Pioneering Studies in C
Neuroscience

Pioneering Studies in Cognitive Neuroscience

Richard A.P. Roche and Seán Commins

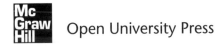
Open University Press

Open University Press
McGraw-Hill Education
McGraw-Hill House
Shoppenhangers Road
Maidenhead
Berkshire
England
SL6 2QL

email: enquiries@openup.co.uk
world wide web: www.openup.co.uk

and

Two Penn Plaza, New York, NY 10121-2289, USA

First published 2009

A catalogue record of this book is available from the British Library

ISBN-13: 978-0-33-523356-4 (pb) 978-0-33-523355-7 (hb)
ISBN-10: 0-33-523356-2 (pb) 0-33-523355-4 (hb)

Library of Congress Cataloging-in-Publication Data
CIP data applied for

Typeset by Graphicraft Ltd, Hong Kong
Printed in the UK by Bell and Bain Ltd, Glasgow.

Fictitious names of companies, products, people, characters and/or data that
may be used herein (in case studies or in examples) are not intended to
represent any real individual, company, product or event.

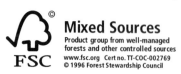

Mixed Sources
Product group from well-managed
forests and other controlled sources
www.fsc.org Cert no. TT-COC-002769
© 1996 Forest Stewardship Council

The McGraw-Hill Companies

Contents

Figures

Tables

Contributors

Charles W. Anderson is Associate Professor in the Department of Computer Science, Colorado State University, Fort Collins, Colorado, USA

Niels Birbaumer is a Professor of Neurology at the Institute of Medical Psychology and Behavioural Neurobiology, Eberhard-Karls-University of Tübingen, Germany

Seán Commins is a Senior Lecturer in Psychology in the Department of Psychology, National University of Ireland Maynooth, Co. Kildare, Ireland

James Danckert is Associate Professor of Psychology at the Department of Psychology, University of Waterloo, Ontario, Canada

Beatrice de Gelder is a Professor of Philosophy and Psychology at the Massachussets General Hospital & Harvard Medical School, Charlestown, USA

Paul Dockree is a Postdoctoral Research Fellow at the Trinity College Institute of Neuroscience, University of Dublin, Trinity College, Dublin, Ireland

Luciano Fadiga is a Professor of Neurophysiology at the University of Ferrara, Italy

Gereon Fink is a Professor of Neurology and Director at the Institut für Neurowissenschaften und Biophysik Medizin, Forschungszentrum Julich, Germany

John Foxe is Associate Professor, Program in Cognitive Neuroscience, Nathan Kline Institute for Psychiatric Research, New York, USA

Eleanor Maguire is a Professor of Neurology at the Wellcome Department Cognitive Neurology, Institute of Neurology, London, UK

Shane O'Mara is Associate Professor, School of Psychology and Trinity College Institute of Neuroscience, University of Dublin, Trinity College, Dublin, Ireland

Alvaro Pascual-Leone is a Professor of Neurology in the Department of Neurology, Harvard Medical School, Boston, MA, USA

V.S. Ramachandran is Director of the Center for Brain and Cognition, and Professor in the Psychology Department at the University of California, San Diego, USA

Lynn Robertson is Adjunct Professor in Neurology and Director of the Cognitive Neuropsychology Laboratory, University of Berkeley, California, USA

Richard A.P. Roche is a Lecturer in Psychology in the Department of Psychology, National University of Ireland Maynooth, Co. Kildare, Ireland

Giuseppe Vallar is a Professor of Physiological Psychology at the University of Milano-Bicocca, Milan, Italy

Vincent Walsh is Professor of Human Brain Research and Reader in Psychology at the Institute of Cognitive Neuroscience, University College London, London, UK

1 Cognitive neuroscience: introduction and historical perspective

Richard A.P. Roche, Seán Commins and Paul M. Dockree

Foreword

The brain is life's most magnificent enigma. Nestling snugly inside the skull sits the most complex object anyone will ever know. The seat of all intelligence, creativity, hope, faith, desire, rage, genius, joy and despair, this grey lump of tissue hides its secrets in deep, shadowy crevices and shiny protrusions. Roughly the weight of a bag of sugar, partially hollow and composed of three-quarters water, one hundred billion cells cling together in its wet darkness, clasping hands and whispering messages to their neighbours. And in this constant chatter of neurons, the electric hum of signals sent in milliseconds, that fathomless universe behind the eyes can generate more thoughts than there are atoms in all of creation.

It is a greedy organ; it demands 20 per cent of the body's blood and oxygen supply to carry out its myriad functions. It can repair itself to a remarkable extent when damaged, as cells grow new connections to bridge the gaps in broken processing chains. It contains many paradoxes, being simultaneously ugly in form and yet strangely elegant. It is malleable – rewiring its physical structure with every new experience – but also stubborn: connections made in childhood can last until old age. It has given rise to the most sublime art and the most monstrous atrocities. It produces a unique personality for every individual on the planet, and can store a lifetime's worth of memories for each person. It is the most elaborate processing system that has ever existed, and is, itself, the reason that we can know this.

In this light, the challenge of unravelling the mysteries of the human brain seems daunting. But despite this, it is widely acknowledged that we have learned more in the past 50 years about the workings of the brain than we managed in the previous two thousand. Pivotal advances in technology, anatomy and physiology, coupled with the study of remarkable individuals with specific brain injury, and the application of cognitive psychological frameworks have led to the emergence of cognitive neuroscience, a discipline dedicated to the brain and its study. We are, therefore, better equipped now than at any other time in human history in our attempts to understand how the brain accomplishes such staggering feats of processing and computation. In this book, we highlight some of the most innovative, original and creative studies in cognitive neuroscience from the last 20 years, and in so doing provide an insight into the process of research, and how some of the brain's most closely guarded secrets can sometimes be teased from it with a clever or unorthodox approach. Given that it is, after all, the brain that is under investigation, to emphasize the creativity of these studies seems somehow appropriate.

Organization of the book

Each and every experimental study carried out in science is a story in itself; it contains a beginning, middle and end, it involves characters and relationships, it has a plot that sometimes twists and turns until an unexpected revelation is reached. This book tells the story of seven recent experiments in cognitive neuroscience which, though drawn from different areas within the field, are all remarkable for the same reason: they demonstrate an innovative approach, an ingenious design and an important finding in that area of research. These studies span each of the major sub-disciplines within cognitive neuroscience, including vision, attention, memory, motor systems, voluntary action, emotion, plasticity and multisensory integration. By discussing these studies, we illustrate what constitutes a clever or ground-breaking experimental design in cognitive neuroscience, and convey the scope for creativity that exists in the process of experimental design.

Each chapter begins with a brief background and description of the study, including an overview of the methodology used and a summary of results. In the next section, one of the principal authors of the study provides a brief commentary on the experiment, the genesis of the idea, the impact the study had and its subsequent implications in that area of research. In the final section of each chapter, a peer expert in the same area of research gives an additional testimonial as to the ingenuity and impact of the study, how it advanced research in the area and the influence it has had on their own experimental designs and ways of thinking about the discipline. The objective of this book is to provide a collection of unique, innovative and significant examples of high-quality research carried out in cognitive neuroscience in recent years. The intention is to provide and foster a sense of enthusiasm and appreciation for the intelligence of the designs used and the significant application and dedication involved in generating the selected pieces of research. In some cases this even extends to the friendships formed and collaborations initiated by the authors, or the memorable patients involved in some of these studies and their own unique stories. We hope that, by telling the story of these seven studies, we provide the reader with a range of insights into the mechanics of carrying out research within science at large, and within cognitive neuroscience specifically.

Historical introduction

No discipline is born fully formed. It will often evolve from something quite different, being shaped by factors like preceding trends, economic/political concerns or the 'received wisdom' of the day. Chance and coincidence frequently play a major role in the genesis of a field of study, and an isolated event can steer the direction of a discipline as surely as a bank of hard rock will divert the course of a river. At the most basic level of analysis, the development of any academic area of study is invariably the story of some remarkable individuals. Perhaps nowhere is this more accurate than in the emergence of cognitive neuroscience, where fascinating patients with rare brain injuries have been as pivotal (arguably more pivotal in some cases) as the scientists who studied them – Pierre Paul Broca is rarely mentioned without quick reference to his patient 'Tan', while the names of H.M. and Brenda Milner are now almost inextricably linked. The next section provides a brief history of the development of cognitive neuroscience, from the earliest written references to the brain, via a number of remarkable individuals (both patients and scientists) to the convergence of theory and technology that brought about the naming of the discipline in the back of a New York taxi cab at the end of the 1970s.

Early references

The search for the earliest references to the brain takes us back as far as one of the first human civilizations, the Sumerians. By 4000 BC, this small tribal culture had grown into a fully fledged society, developing in the rich crop-growing lands at the confluence of the rivers Tigris and Euphrates, a tract of land dubbed the Fertile Crescent. Aside from forming an impressive agricultural society, developing what may be the world's first written language (a system of hieroglyphs that may predate that of the ancient Egyptians) and producing the most important invention of all, the wheel, it appears that the Sumerians were also the first society to engage in recreational drug use. A stone tablet of text dating from this period describes the consequences of ingesting the poppy plant from which, of course, opium is derived. The text describes in exquisite detail the euphoric mind-altering effects of the drug on its user, and constitutes the earliest reference to the mind/brain yet discovered.

More clues that early cultures viewed the brain (or at least the head) of great importance to life and well-being come from the discovery of skulls bearing large and intentionally drilled holes. This process of trepanning or trepanation appears to have been common in many societies (including pre-Incan cultures in South America) around 2000 BC. Crude surgical implements were used to drill holes directly into the skull of seemingly willing individuals, with some variation in the size and location of the 'surgery'. It is likely that the process served some spiritual function, perhaps aiding the release of spirits from the brain, while some argue that it represents an early medical intervention. It is worth remembering that in many non-western societies today, these two different needs are in fact considered one and the same. Explanations aside, we can only guess at some of the damage to the brain's surface that must have resulted from these crude operations, and at the symptoms of such damage.

The first case study of a person suffering from brain injury originates in ancient Egypt. The document, a papyrus scroll that has been dated to *c.* 1700 BC, has become known as the Edwin Smith Surgical Papyrus after the man who fortuitously became its owner. Smith was an American Egyptologist and collector of antiquities. While meandering through a street market in Luxor in 1862, Smith bought a tattered papyrus scroll from a street vendor for a modest fee. When the hieroglyphics were subsequently deciphered by James Henry Breadstead (assisted by the physiologist Arno Luckhardt), it became apparent that Smith had unwittingly obtained one of the most important documents in medical history. The text consisted of a succession of medical case studies, each described in rigorous detail and vivid clarity. And most significantly, of the 48 case studies listed, 27 gave accounts of head or brain injuries. It is in these yellowed and sun-bleached pages that the first written description of the brain in the human record can be found. In fact, the case studies go so far as to describe the convolutions of the brain's surface (referring to them as 'corrugations'), the meninges ('membrane enveloping the brain') and even cerebrospinal fluid.

The ancient Greeks were the next civilization to consider the question of the mind, and prominent philosophers such as Aristotle and Alcmaeon were among those to ponder the issues of mind, soul and psyche (terms that they often used interchangeably). Terminology aside, the great thinkers of the day had agreed on the existence of some ethereal driving force that is responsible for the behaviour of the body, a concept later adopted by Christianity. While some had argued that the heart was the central organ for thought and sensation, Alcmaeon (450 BC) concluded that the brain, rather than the heart, was the seat of the mind. Plato (427–437 BC) was also of the opinion that the brain was the home of mental processes, a view not shared by his most famous student, Aristotle (384–322 BC). Aristotle went on to suggest that the heart was the source of the mind, producing all emotions and thoughts, like a furnace, and the role of the brain was akin to that of a radiator, to simply cool the heart down. With Aristotle, we see the beginnings of a dualistic view of mind and brain, a separation of the material and non-material, which would surface again later in the history of neuroscience with the theory of Descartes.

While the Greek philosophers were grappling with the nature of the mind, and its relation to the body, the ancient Alexandrians were taking a more pragmatic approach by dissecting human cadavers and comparing the anatomy to that of other animals. Such early pioneers included Herophilus (335–280 BC) and Erasistratus (304–250 BC), who carried out detailed investigations of the major organs. Their studies of the brain and the heart led them to agree with Alcmaeon and Plato, concluding that intelligence could be localized to the ventricles of the brain due to their larger size in humans relative to other mammals. Furthermore, they were the first to discover and describe the nervous system, classifying nerve cells into two types, sensory and motor.

The Renaissance to phrenology (1500–1800 AD)

Due largely to the rapid spread of Christianity and the resultant ban on human dissection imposed by the Church, relatively few advances were made in the study of the brain from the period 280 BC to c. AD 1500. The handful of notable exceptions during this fallow period for brain science include Galen's lecture 'On the Brain' in AD 177, the description of surgical procedures for neurological disorders by Al-Zahrawi (or Albucasis) around AD 1000, the publication of Mondino de'Luzzi's anatomy textbook, *Anothomia*, in 1316 and the opening of hospitals exclusively for the mentally ill, St Mary of Bethlehem in 1402 and in Valencia in 1410. Throughout this period, primitive brain surgery would often take place in secret, as unskilled physicians (often enterprising barbers) carried out clandestine procedures to remove the 'stone of madness', the biological cause of an invalid's malady. The relative inactivity in neuroscience research during this large historical epoch is balanced by the explosion in such investigation that coincided with the beginning of the Renaissance in Italy around 1500. From the early years of the sixteenth century, the study of the workings of both brain and body grew at a phenomenal rate, with one of the earliest studies carried out by Leonardo da Vinci himself – a wax cast of the human ventricles, produced in 1504.

Over the course of the next 200 years, a succession of significant advances were made, including the publication of the first neuroscience textbook *De Humani Corporis* by Vesalius in 1543, Pratensis' book on neurological disorder *De Cerebri Morbis* in 1549, the description of hydrocephalus by Vesalius in 1550, the coining of the term 'hippocampus' by Giulio Cesare Aranzi in 1564, the identification of white matter by Piccolomini in 1583 and the description of the lateral (or Sylvian) fissure of the brain in 1641 by Francisco de la Boe Sylvius. Major progress was also made during this period in the understanding of the visual system and its workings, while research was also beginning into such biologically based problems as depression (Robert Burton published *The Anatomy of Melancholy* in 1621), stroke (Johann Jakof Wepfer suggested the role of broken blood vessels in stroke in 1658) and meningitis (Thomas Willis published a case study of this disorder in 1661). Willis also published *Cerebri Anatome* in 1664, and was to coin the term 'neurology' in 1681.

One of the most prominent figures from this time was the French philosopher, mathematician and physiologist René Descartes (1596–1650), who was particularly interested in how the brain might play a role in the execution of behaviour. Having seen an automated mannequin of St Germaine, which was controlled by liquid being pumped through hollow tubes running throughout the statue, he proposed that nerve cells operated in a comparable manner. He theorized that 'animal spirits' coursed through the nervous system, with nerves acting like hollow tubes that allowed these spirits to flow towards particular muscles. Most significantly, Descartes viewed the relationship between mind and brain as *dualistic*; he considered the mind and the body as separate entities, independent but also interconnected. He viewed the pineal gland as the point at which the non-material mind interacted with the material brain. While his conception of the operation of nerves has since been shown to be inaccurate, his emphasis on the pineal gland misplaced, and his dualistic standpoint logically untenable, the impact of Descartes on the history of neuroscience is still noteworthy: his proposal that a non-material mind is controlling the physical body is one of the most influential ideas to emerge from this period. In attempting to understand how these two entities might interact, he coined the mind–body problem, a question that has resulted in a vast amount of philosophical discussion and experimental investigation in our attempts to understand it.

Interest in the brain and nervous system continued throughout the eighteenth century, and more breakthroughs followed. Important insights were gained into such topics as reflexes (by Jean Astruc in 1736), the cranial nerves (von Soemmerring described the 12 cranial nerves in 1778), cerebrospinal fluid (von Haller's description from 1766) and the addictive properties of alcohol (Benjamin Rush in 1784). Some ideas from this period were to find considerable longevity – Hartley was the first to use the term 'psychology' in 1749; Le Roy pioneered the use of electroconvulsive therapy for mental disorders in 1755 – while others would meet with less widespread scientific support over the coming centuries – Anton Mesmer embarked on his study of animal magnetism, which would evolve into hypnotism, in 1774. As a result of this intense

interest in physiology, progress in brain anatomy and advances in scientific measurement techniques, a good deal was known about the physical structure, if not the
mechanisms, of the human brain by the beginning of the nineteenth century. This
was to culminate in the first organized attempt to relate brain structure (even if by
proxy) to behaviour and personality in the form of phrenology.

Phrenology was proposed originally by Franz Joseph Gall (1758–1828) in 1808, but
his early writings on the subject were little more than anecdotes; Gall described how
acquaintances of his displayed an aptitude for a particular capacity such as memory,
and he related this capacity to any prominent physical feature of the head that he
could identify – bulging eyes, for example, suggested to Gall that the brain behind the
eye area was enlarged, and therefore related to this enhanced cognitive function. It was
through Gall's collaborations with Johann Spurzheim (1776–1832) that phrenology
began to take the form of a scientific discipline. Together, Gall and Spurzheim developed
a technique whereby the bumps and contours of the human skull could be measured,
and any protrusions or recesses on the skull surface could be associated with particular
mental faculties or personality traits that were notable in that person. Through this
process, a map of the head was developed showing 35 separate sections, each associated
with a personality trait such as 'language', 'romantic love', 'logic' or 'humility'. A bump
or protrusion of one of these areas suggested that the underlying area of the brain was
enlarged, and had pushed that section of skull outwards, revealing an enhancement of
that capacity. Some of the faculties identified on such maps were remarkably abstract,
with some phrenology busts from the era identifying capacities such as 'preference for
solids' and 'love of the magnificent'.

While phrenology was soon to be discredited, and has since become a topic of
humour in modern culture, elements of the theory are largely consistent with aspects
of contemporary neuroscience. At its heart, phrenology was presenting a *localizationist*
view of the brain – it proposed that particular mental functions (language, memory,
vision, etc.) were associated with discrete areas of the brain and not with other areas,
an assumption still fundamental to the neuroscientists' credo today. Unfortunately
for Gall, Spurzheim and their followers, the assumption that larger brain regions led to
protrusions on the surface of the skull was unfounded. Without access to the type of
neuroimaging techniques available now, the only means the phrenologists had of
carrying out objective, scientific measurements was to examine the surface of the
skull. They were doing the best they could with the technology available to them at
the time, and it was this reliance on the exterior of the skull that led them to their
inaccurate assumption, and ultimately, to ridicule.

The holist–localist debate

While the phrenologists were promoting their slightly skewed version of localizationism,
the respected French biologist Pierre Flourens (1794–1867) was conducting experiments on the brains of dogs, rabbits and birds that were leading him to a different
conclusion about how the brain worked. He repeatedly carried out lesion studies in
these animals and observed similar patterns of preserved cognitive functions in the
creatures, irrespective of where the lesion was located. When he carried out small and
discrete lesions, he often saw little or no change to the behaviour of the animal. On the

other hand, when he carried out large-scale ablations of huge sections of cortex, the animal was typically incapable of any behaviour, even simple responses to stimuli. He took this as in indication that function could not be localized to particular regions of the cortex, but rather the whole brain is involved in every mental process, which he termed the brain's *aggregate field*. He championed this *holistic* or *globalistic* view of the brain, and in so doing, sounded the death knell for phrenology. He claimed the demonstration of such a dramatic recovery of function in his experimental animals was conclusive evidence against a localizationist view; if the remaining undamaged parts of cortex can compensate for and carry out the functions of the damaged regions, he claimed, then *all of the brain* must be capable of carrying out *all of these processes*. While his reasoning seems sound, we now know that Flourens had seriously under-estimated the amazing capacity of the brain to recover from damage, the highly plastic nature of its structure and the versatility of neurons to adapt to new situations. While the globalist–holist viewpoint enjoyed brief popularity and acceptance (due in part to the eminence of Flourens himself), and played a crucial role in the history of neuroscience by ending the popularity of phrenology, several case studies of neuro-logical damage were soon to appear that would tilt the balance of favour firmly back towards the localizationist camp.

John Hughlings Jackson (1835–1911), a physician who treated patients suffering from epilepsy, began to notice some common patterns in the behaviour of his patients when they were having a seizure. He observed how, as the attack progressed, the spasms and trembling would follow a similar bodily route, affecting first the extremities, then the rest of the limbs and moving on to the torso. This commonality suggested to Jackson that, as excitation spread across the brain during an epileptic fit, the parts of the body governed by those brain regions responded by showing seizure activity. He was effectively proposing a topographic organization of the cortex, in which the legs were controlled by sets of cells in a distinct part of the brain, the arms in another region, and so on. We now know, from mapping the motor and sensory cortices and the bodily maps contained therein, that he was correct, and that the motor and sensory cortices are indeed organized topographically. Jackson's brand of localizationism was a major blow to the globalist standpoint, but further case studies of brain injury reported by Paul Broca and Karl Wernicke were to prove the twin nails in the coffin of globalism.

Pierre Paul Broca (1824–1880), a French physician with a particular interest in patients suffering from brain injury, was presented in 1861 with a most unusual case. The patient, who had suffered a stroke in the left hemisphere, was unable to generate coherent speech; he was capable of understanding language, and could read and write, but his speech production was limited to simple, nonsense utterances such as 'Tan'. After 'Tan's' death, examination of his brain revealed that his aphasia was the result of damage to a portion of the left frontal cortex now referred to as Broca's Area. This represented a dramatic demonstration of a specific cognitive capacity – the ability to generate speech – being localized to a discrete region of the cortex, while other, related capacities – language comprehension – remained unaffected, presumably because it was located in a separate area of the brain. With globalism falling out of favour thanks to the observations of Jackson, all that was missing was a complementary case study showing the reverse pattern for localizationism to become installed as the accepted view on brain function. Such a case study was to arrive 15 years later. In 1876, another stroke patient presented with a different set of symptoms – he was capable of speech, but what he produced made no sense. Here was a double dissociation with the case of Tan, who could understand language but not produce it. The case was reported by the German physician Karl Wernicke (1848–1904), and on posthumous examination of the patient's brain, the region of damage – an area near the left temporoparietal junction – was dubbed Wernicke's area.

Meanwhile in America, a freak accident had transformed a previously unassuming railroad worker into one of the most famous case studies in the history of neuroscience. Phineas Gage (1823–1860) was a foreman working on the construction of the railroad in Vermont. His particular responsibility was to oversee the removal of large outcroppings of rock from the path of the rail track, a task that was accomplished by drilling a hole deep into the rock, filling the resultant crevice with explosive powder and blasting the obstruction out. Gage's role was to use a special tamping iron, a metal rod of his own design measuring over $3^1/2$ feet long and $1^1/4$ inches in diameter, to push or 'tamp' the explosives into the centre of the boulder or rock. Typically, sand would be poured on top of the explosive powder to reduce the risk of igniting it via a spark, but the job was still a very dangerous occupation. On a fateful afternoon in September 1848, Gage, momentarily distracted, began to tamp down the explosive powder before the sand had been added. The subsequent impact of iron on rock produced a spark that ignited the gunpowder in a sudden explosion, driving the tamping iron through Gage's head. The rod entered Gage below his left cheekbone, travelling upwards, and exited via the top of his head, removing with it large portions of his prefrontal cortex. The force of the explosion was so great that the rod was found almost 100 metres away. Remarkably, Gage survived this trauma, and having fended off a severe infection as a result of his injury, appeared to have made a full recovery. However, as his physician Dr J.M. Harlow was to observe, Gage's personality appeared significantly altered by the experience. What had previously been an efficient, mannerly and well-liked young man had become, in Harlow's words, 'fitful, irreverent, indulging at times in the grossest profanity'. In addition, his behaviour was disinhibited, unpredictable and disorganized, engaging in the formation of multiple outlandish plans that were rapidly abandoned in favour of new ones.

While the extent of the change in Gage's personality appears to have been exaggerated by some later accounts (in some versions of the story he became a drunkard and gambler, involved in brawls and other loutish behaviour), what is undisputed is the fact that Gage underwent a significant alteration of his mental faculties and personality as a result of his loss of brain tissue. By the time of his death in 1860, his fame had already begun following a stint as a sideshow attraction (complete with his tamping iron) in P.T. Barnum's museum, but Gage's true legacy goes far beyond that of a curio in a freakshow; his impact on the development of cognitive neuroscience has ensured him a more enduring type of fame as one of the most important case studies in the history of brain science.

Faced with such compelling evidence for the localisationist perspective, the holist view crumbled. Further support for localism was to follow in the 1870s, when Gustav Fritsch (1838–1907) and Eduard Hitzig (1838–1927) carried out experiments involving the electrical stimulation of the motor cortex of dogs. They found that stimulation of particular areas of motor cortex would cause different parts of the animal – neck, hind legs, forelegs – to twitch. In 1909, Korbinian Brodmann (1868–1918) published a map of the brain that had been divided in 52 different areas based not on associated behaviours or personality traits, as the phrenologists had done, but rather on the types of neural cells present in each. He was a noted histologist, and had studied the different cell types in the brain, with particular interest in how they were distributed in the cortex. His cytoarchitechtonic map of the cortex lent more support to the localizationist view, as implicit in this map was the idea that cells with different physical structures may serve different functions. Nearly 100 years after its publication, the use of Brodmann's areas to describe the location of an area of cortex is still a convention in modern cognitive neuroscience.

Modern pioneers

The twentieth century saw neuroscience come of age. At the start of the last century, the discipline was self-consciously ill-defined, with elements of anatomy and physiology awkwardly juxtaposed with psychology and medicine, as well as a somewhat nervous nod towards philosophy. By the close of the 1990s, however, this clumsy adolescent had grown into a confident and fully formed field of study in its own right, proudly leading the way into a new millennium shoulder to shoulder with the more venerable sciences. This transformation came about due to a number of factors; several significant discoveries were made in the first half of the twentieth century, and the latter half saw the convergence of related fields like cognitive psychology, computational modelling and clinical neuropsychology with advances in brain imaging and electrical/magnetic recording techniques. This fusion of interests and approaches resulted in the naming of a new discipline, 'cognitive neuroscience', in the late 1970s, and it is the emergence of this new discipline that we will delineate in this section. We begin by returning to the early years of the last century.

Around the same time as Brodmann was compiling his map of the cortex, Santiago Ramon y Cajal (1852–1934) and Camillo Golgi (1843–1956) were on the verge of sharing the Nobel Prize (in 1906) for their work on visualizing neurons. Cajal was a Spanish anatomist who came to study the structure of the nervous system following his original training as a medic and then a period in the army. While pursuing this interest in anatomy at the University of Madrid, he was introduced in 1887 to the technique of silver staining tissue slices, a method that had been pioneered by Golgi over a decade before. Applying these staining techniques to his samples of neural tissue, Cajal was stunned by the clarity with which the nerve cells became visible under his microscope. Here, Cajal's talent for drawing was to prove important (he had originally planned to be an artist), as he produced exquisitely detailed diagrams of the cell structures he was now able to observe. The most important discovery to emerge from this work was the realization that the brain and nervous system did not consist of a continuous mass of cytoplasm, as most (including Golgi[1]) believed up to this point. His neuron doctrine would state this fact, along with the idea that neurons were the primary functional unit of the brain, the identification of synapses as the spaces between them, and the polar nature of neural cells.

Among the other key figures of the early twentieth century are Johannes Evangelista Purkinje (1787–1869), who was the first to provide a detailed description of the cells that now bear his name, Hans Berger (1873–1941), who was the first to record the electrical activity of the human brain from the scalp in 1929, giving birth to the study of the human electroencephalogram (or electrocephalography – EEG), and Karl Lashley (1890–1958), who spent his career in search of the 'engram' – the cortical basis of a memory – by carrying out a systematic (and ultimately fruitless) series of lesions to the brains of rats in an attempt to sever the biological substrates of the links that learning had wrought. Another milestone came in 1932, when Sir Charles Sherrington (1857–1952) won the Nobel Prize for his work on the synapse, shifting the level of analysis from the neuron to the synapse as the key locus of cellular communication. In 1949, the great Canadian biologist Donal Hebb (1904–1985) was to outline his theory of the rules that might govern changes in cellular connectivity – Hebb's law. This description was to prove startlingly apt when the phenomenon of long-term potentiation (LTP) was described in 1973 by Bliss and Lomo, a mechanism that remains the most compelling model of how memories are represented on a cellular level.

Throughout the 1950s, Wilder Penfield (1891–1976) pioneered neurosurgical techniques, and discovered that the application of electrical pulses to the surface of the cortex could produce specific reactions – sensations, vocalizations, memories – in an awake patient. His findings were to have a profound impact on the development of modern neuroscience. Also in the 1950s, a young Canadian who would become known as Patient H.M. underwent surgery for severe intractable epilepsy – the bilateral removal of his hippocampi and amygdalae would be a success in terms of stopping his seizures, but he would be left with a form of anterograde amnesia that would prevent him from learning and retaining any new factual information for the rest of his life. The study of H.M.'s deficits (and preserved functions) has provided insights into the operation of the memory system that eclipse all that had been discovered in the previous two millennia, and have imbued H.M. with the dubious honour of being the most studied human being in medical history.

In the wake of these and other landmarks, the study of the brain gained significant momentum, and by the late 1970s, a name was required to encompass the many different strands of research that were beginning to converge in this attempt to unravel the mysteries of the brain. Cognitive psychology, which had become dominant since behaviourism fell out of favour in the 1950s, had provided this new discipline with useful cognitive models and experimental methods for studying cognition in humans. Experimental and clinical neuropsychology was beginning to reveal much about cognitive processes and their neural underpinnings via the study of patients who had suffered brain injuries and other neurological damage. Advances in radiography and EEG techniques now allowed both the metabolic and electrical activity of the brain to be observed while a conscious participant engaged in a particular cognitive task, for the first time allowing both the spatial and temporal aspects of cortical processing to be delineated. And developments in computing applications had seen the advent of computer models that could mimic the activity of neural networks and brain structures. All these disciplines appeared to be moving towards a common destination – they were asking similar or complementary questions about the nature of the brain, and each one provided novel routes to the answers. The formal birth of the discipline of cognitive neuroscience occurred in 1979, as two leading lights of this new field, Michael Gazzaniga and George Miller, shared a taxi to a dinner held in New York to discuss this new area of research. The pair, realizing that the field was as yet formally unchristened, settled on the moniker 'cognitive neuroscience', and introduced it at the subsequent dinner. The term stuck, and while this is undoubtedly not the first case of a birth taking place in the rear of a New York taxi cab, history may look back on it as being among the most significant.

Tools of the trade

Today, the discipline has not only an accepted name, but it also boasts a wide variety of methodological approaches and techniques that allow contemporary cognitive neuroscientists to investigate whatever aspect of brain function and cognitive processing they select. These techniques represent a veritable arsenal of tools at our disposal, ranging from indices of brain metabolism and electrical activity to lesion approaches in both human and animal. In the final section of this chapter, we briefly describe the main approaches used in modern cognitive neuroscience, with particular emphasis on the techniques that are used in the seven pioneering studies, which are discussed in the remainder of this book.

Position emission tomography (PET), functional magnetic resonance imaging (MRI) and brain imaging techniques

The possibility of measuring a reliable physiological correlate of neural activity in a non-invasive fashion has long been the hope of psychologists. The ambition of Wilhelm Wündt, who first brought psychology into the laboratory, was to investigate the physiological conditions of conscious events, but his reliance on behavioural correlates of introspective experiences fell short of providing a window into the mind. Nevertheless, an important discovery emerged during Wundt's tenure that would transform to field of *physiological psychology* into *cognitive neuroscience* one hundred years later: Roy and Sherrington (1890) established that when neurons are active they consume oxygen carried by haemoglobin in red blood cells; thus an increase in neural activity in a particular brain area is fuelled by blood flow to that region to supply oxygen. In 1990 Seiji Ogawa recognized the considerable importance of blood oxygen level as a correlate of neural activity that is detectable through functional magnetic resonance imaging (fMRI) (Ogawa et al., 1990) and two years later Kwong and colleagues were the first to use fMRI to measure brain activity in human participants (Kwong et al., 1992).

Functional imaging relies on the haemodynamic response, which is the relative difference between high levels of oxygenated blood supplying *active* neurons versus low oxyhemoglobin uptake for *inactive* neurons; this difference yields variation in magnetic receptiveness to oxyhemoglobin and deoxyhemoglobin, providing a magnetic signal detectable in an MRI scanner. This form of MRI is known as blood oxygenation level dependent (BOLD) imaging and is the most commonly used approach. Typically, fMRI is used to produce activation maps depicting which parts of the brain are involved in a particular mental process. It should be stressed that fMRI relies on the emergence of statistical trends across many trials; thus, a single perceptual event, cognitive process or action will not produce a reliable activation map on its own. Experimental stimuli are repeatedly presented to a participant to determine the areas of the brain that reliably produce to magnetic signal variation.

Functional imaging provides an invaluable tool to capture dynamic changes in brain function but its utility extends beyond this: diffusion tensor imaging (DTI) uses MRI technology to detect the direction and magnitude of water diffusion through cellular tissues in the brain. Water movement is constrained by the organization of white matter fibres that serve as communication channels interconnecting the brain's information processing grey matter. Poor cognitive function, age-related decline and debilitating illnesses such as multiple sclerosis (MS) are related to deterioration in the structure and integrity of the white matter tracts and DTI provides an important means to measure the effectiveness of all these important communication channels in the brain.

PET is an older imaging technique than fMRI. It uses radioactive substances that are injected into the human participant to provide images of the brain. Most cognitive neuroscience studies are conducted with H_2 ^{15}O labelled water via an intravenous injection. The radioisotope is absorbed throughout the physical matter of the body, and the regions of brain with the highest blood flow will have increased concentrations of this radioactive oxygen. The radioactive isotopes emit positrons that collide with electrons, emitting two photons (gamma rays). A ring of detector units in the scanner surrounding the brain receive gamma rays and these data are used to construct a map of radioactivities that indicate the relative levels of activation across different brain regions. The main limitation of PET, in contrast to fMRI, is its ability to detect fast-evolving perceptual or cognitive changes and therefore reduce the type of psychological experience that is amenable to investigation. A general limitation applying to both PET and fMRI research is that they are restricted at the physiological level in how we should interpret a region of 'activation'. It is unknown whether a pattern of activation reflects excitatory or inhibition neural transmission (Buckner and Logan, 2001) that constrains our interpretation in terms of the nature of interactions across neural networks.

Human EEG, ERPs and source dipole analysis

Whereas functional MRI has high spatial resolution (in the region of 3–6 millimetres), it has relatively poor temporal resolution (the hemodynamic response rises to a peak over 4–5 seconds). EEG directly measures the brain's electrical activity, giving high temporal (~milliseconds) but low spatial resolution. The two techniques are therefore complementary in addressing pertinent questions within the field of cognitive neuroscience.

EEG is acquired from 32, 64, 128 or 256 electrodes positioned on different locations on the surface of the scalp. EEG signals (recorded in micro-volts) are amplified and digitalized for later analysis. EEG activity arises from the summation of neural activity; it is not possible to measure the activity from a single dendrite or neuron using this technique (see below for alternatives in non-human animal research). Instead, EEG measures the collective activity of thousands of neurons that are synchronized and represent non-random processes. If this EEG activity were distributed randomly in polarity and in time, the net surface potential would be zero but this is not the case so we can be confident that patterns of physiological activity recorded at this macro level are arising from large coordinated neural networks. However, it is important to recognize the spatial restrictions of EEG. The scalp electrodes primarily detect currents emanating from superficial layers of the cortex, on the crests of gyri directly underlying the skull; the radial arrangements of apical dendrites in the cortex occupy this position. Currents that are not oriented to the scalp are not picked up by the EEG. Thus, neurons buried within the sulci or within deep brain structures have far less contribution to the EEG signal.

EEG provides an ongoing continuous recording of the brain's electrical activity; however, discrete neural signals can be extracted called event-related potentials (ERPs). An ERP signal emerges in response to sensory, perceptual or cognitive events when a participant is engaged in a psychological task. In response to each stimulus presented to the participant, a systematic fluctuation in the EEG signal, characterized by a positive or negative deflection, is recorded. As with functional imaging techniques, it is difficult to identify a robust signal after the presentation of a single stimulus. Consequently, many repetitions of the stimuli are needed to generate an average signal. This technique cancels out noise in the signal allowing only the voltage amplitude (measured in micro-volts) in response to the stimulus to stand out clearly. The ERP technique has proved very useful because the timing and magnitude of these electrical potentials and the location of this activity on the scalp are used to make inferences about the time course of mental processing.

The ERP is extracted from the broadband EEG signal but other techniques can reveal more about electrophysiological correlates of mental activity by decomposing brain rhythms into different frequency bands; for example, theta (3–5 cycles per second) and alpha (c. 10 cycles per second). The prevalence or 'power' of each band can be measured and these are known as 'oscillatory EEG states'. These states have considerable behavioural, physiological and neurochemical relevance: for instance, during periods when individuals are alert and receptive, the alpha rhythm – a key attention-sensitive EEG signal – changes in power (Ray and Cole, 1985).

The limited spatial resolution of EEG can be improved by increasing the number of recording sites during acquisition (Murro et al., 1995) and using mathematical models to estimate the electrical sources of the surface recordings. Ultimately, the current distribution from inside the head cannot be uniquely determined from the electrical field patterns (or scalp topographies) recorded at the scalp. This problem has been described as the inverse problem; nevertheless, different models provide useful, albeit approximate, solutions to this inverse problem. There are many classes of model (Cacioppo et al., 2007) but the most basic technique is the equivalent dipole approach. The equivalent dipole source model makes the assumption that potentials recorded at the surface emerge from a small number of relatively focal sources. The dipole itself does not represent a discrete source but instead a statistical centre of gravity that represents the synchronized activity of a number of neurons (~100,000 pyramidal neurons). The assumptions built into this approach necessarily require the scientist to have a good a priori reason for examining particular neuroanatomical areas (often based on previous functional imaging data or intracranial studies). The parameters included in the typical dipole model are location, orientation and amplitude of the source. Using an iterative fitting procedure the model attempts to use these parameters to explain the greatest variance of the signal waveform recorded at the scalp. Using the equivalent dipole approach it is easier to model signals that emerge nearer to the cortical surface; these reflect localized cortical activity such as visual evoked potentials. By contrast, dipoles originating from deep brain structures are likely part of a broader neural network and are more difficult to account for in the parameters of the model.

Virtual lesions of the human brain – transcranial magnetic stimulation (TMS)

While neuroimaging and electrophysiological approaches can provide a detailed impression of both the areas of activation and the temporal dynamics of such activations during a cognitive task, these techniques are, essentially, correlational in nature. That is, they can reveal the brain areas that are active while a participant performs a particular task, but these may not be the areas that are *necessary* to execute the task. This problem of *functional resolution* is overcome by using the approach of TMS. TMS employs principles based on Faraday's Law that a current can be induced when a conductor is placed within a moving magnetic field (the same principle that allows a bicycle dynamo to work). By placing a large, rapidly changing magnetic field close to the head, the population of neurons in the underlying cortical tissue can be induced to fire in response to this magnetic field change. A current-carrying wire is wound many times into a coil (either circular or figure-eight shape) and placed against the scalp. Passing a large current through the wire generates a strong magnetic field, and by rapidly changing the polarity of this field, the brain cells in the area beneath the coil are caused to fire. This effect has two important uses in neuropsychological research.

First, using single-pulse TMS allows scientists to perform studies similar to the cortical stimulation studies of Penfield and others, but without the necessity of opening up the skull. For example, applying TMS to areas of motor cortex can reveal the extent of cortical tissue that is responsible for controlling the movement of individual fingers. This cortical mapping application of TMS is described in greater detail in Chapter 2. The other research application of TMS is as a *virtual lesion* technique; that is, by inducing cell firing in a population of neurons in response to the external field change, these cells are no longer capable of firing as part of a cortical processing circuit, and are therefore effectively 'knocked out' of that processing loop. In this way, TMS can be said to produce a painless, temporary and reversible lesion of an area of cortex in the human brain while a participant carries out a task. The use of such repetitive-pulse TMS (or rTMS) allows researchers to investigate whether a particular brain region is *required* for a certain cognitive operation to take place, or whether it is merely active at the same time. This use of TMS is discussed in Chapter 8.

The study of humans with brain injury

A patient referred to a neuropsychologist with focal damage in one area of the brain reveals an answer to an important question: is the lesioned area *absolutely* required in a processing chain for a given behaviour? Cognitive neuroscientists can only be definitively sure of the causal relevance of a particular brain structure for behaviour through its damage or absence; functional imaging highlights brain areas that are *correlated* with a given behaviour and not whether they are *causal* for behavioural outcome. The classic case studies by Paul Broca and Karl Wernicke in the nineteenth century illustrate the gold standard of neuropsychological research for understanding functionally independent processes in the brain: the double dissociation. These case studies have been described in detail above. The logic of the double dissociation between the two patients is expressed as follows: function X (articulation of speech) depends on area A (Broca's area) but not area B (Wernicke's area), whereas function Y (comprehending speech) depends on area B (Wernicke's area) but not area A (Broca's area). Therefore, each function operates independently of the other and is mediated by an area with an input and an output to the rest of the system that is independent of the inputs and ouputs of the other area and its associated function. In contemporary research, lesion analysis complements functional imaging by identifying indispensable components of the processing chain. Moreover, functional imaging complements lesion analysis by elucidating the broader network that comprises the processing chain.

Further understanding of brain lesions and their functional role is central for targeted rehabilitation of function and the guided recovery of patients. For instance, in the circumstances of mild to moderate brain injury the underlying brain networks supporting behaviour may have the potential for restoration if an appropriate rehabilitation schedule is adhered to. Self-repair occurs through synaptic turnover, changes in the dendritic branches of neurons with associated changes in the pattern of synaptic connectivity. If two neurons or groups of neurons have been disconnected they may become reconnected if they are repeatedly activated at the same time, conforming to the Hebbian learning principle that 'cells that the fire together wire together' (Hebb, 1949). This principle has guided research to foster adaptive connections within a lesioned network and to minimize the possibility of accidently fostering faulty connections with other networks. For example, Taub et al. (1993) investigated patients who suffered unilateral strokes leading to poor function of one upper limb. They discouraged patients from using their good limb by instructing them to keep their good hand at rest in their pocket and encouraged use of dysfunctional limb. There were significant improvements in motor function after two weeks, lasting up to two years following training. Therefore, the best pattern of stimulation was activation of one limb combined with deactivation of the other.

By contrast, if extensive lesions destroy a large proportion of cells and connections such that circuits cannot recover, the best course of rehabilitative action is compensation and functional reorganization of the system. There is evidence that cortical maps can be modified with experience (see Chapter 2) by altering the demands of the system through increased use. Consequently, cortical areas surrounding the damaged site take over the function. This functional plasticity of the adult cortex demonstrates that brains have built-in damage resistance after injury.

Animal lesion studies

One of the oldest methods used in neuroscience is the lesion technique. In research, a lesion refers to the destruction or removal of a particular region in the brain. This destruction could be accidental, resulting from cell death/loss in a particular area following head injury, cerebrovascular accident or neurodegenerative disease among other causes. Such accidental lesions tend not to be hugely informative due to the inability to control the location of the damaged site or the extent of damage.

Alternatively, the lesion could be intentional whereby a region is surgically removed. Intentional lesions are usually performed on animal subjects; however, in cases of severe epilepsy or brain tumours, removal of brain tissue in humans can be performed. Neuroscientists and neurosurgeons can exercise greater control over such lesions, thereby allowing for the assessment of subsequent behavioural deficits in the subject/participant.

The main lesion techniques include aspiration, electrolytic, neurotoxic and cryo-blockade. The aspiration lesion involves a small suction pump being lowered into the region of interest and tissue is then removed. This method is usually used for cortical rather than subcortical structures. The major disadvantage of the aspiration lesion is that it destroys both the cell bodies of the neurons in the targeted region and also the fibres of passage. Therefore interpretation of any resulting behavioural deficit is difficult due to the inability to distinguish between the destruction of the region itself and the severing of connections between two other areas. An electrolytic lesion can be performed whereby a small electrode is lowered to a specific brain region and a high frequency current is then passed through the electrode tip, which in turn destroys the neurons. The advantage of this technique is that it can be used subcortically; however, like the aspiration lesion, it too destroys the fibres of passage.

Increasingly in research, neurotoxic lesions are used. Here a small cannula is slowly inserted in the targeted region and a neurotoxic substance is released. Such substances include kainic acid, ibotenic acid or the glutamate agonist NMDA. This technique preserves the fibres of passage and can be used to target both cortical and subcortical structures. With cryoblockade lesions a small cryoprobe is inserted and the targeted area is cooled. The advantage of this technique is that the lesions are reversible. Finally, a newly developed method of lesion has been used; this is referred to as the gene knockout or gene knockdown method. Specific genes can be completely deleted or made silent, thereby allowing the effects of these genes on biochemistry, physiology and behaviour (or rather the effects of their absence) to be examined. However, it should be noted that most behavioural traits are as a result of many interacting genes, and also that many genes are influenced by the expression of other genes. Therefore, the behavioural deficits observed following such techniques are often difficult to interpret.

Invasive EEG and single-cell recordings from the awake, freely-moving animal

Both scalp-recorded and invasive EEG can be obtained from the freely-moving animal. Cortical EEG is often recorded through stainless steel skull screws. Subcortical recordings are made through the insertion of an electrode into a targeted brain region. However, these gross-recoded activities are often very difficult to relate to ongoing behaviour and to the activity of singe cells/groups of cells; therefore interpretation of EEG signals can be complex.

Another technique that has proved very useful in determining the activity of a particular brain region is single-cell recording from the awake animal as it performs a particular task. Using this technique it is possible to record action potentials from a single neuron through the use of a microelectrode whose tip is located in the extracellular fluid beside that neuron. Therefore, when the neuron fires an action potential, the electrical discharge is recorded by the electrode and subsequently amplified. This method has been very useful in allowing neuroscientists to record, for example, 'place cells' from the hippocampal region of the rat brain. Place cells are neurons that fire when an animal is in a certain location (O'Keefe and Dostrovsky, 1971). Other cells recorded using such a method include 'head-direction' cells (Taube et al., 1990) and 'grid cells' (e.g. Hafting et al., 2008) in the rat; cells related to visual activity have been recoded from the cat (e.g. Hubel and Wiesel, 1962), including simple cells, orientation cells and complex cells. In addition, 'mirror neurons' (see Chapter 3), 'view responsive' cells (O'Mara et al., 1994) and 'face cells' (e.g. Perrett et al., 1982) have been recorded from the monkey. Interestingly, 'place cells' have also been recoded from the human medial temporal lobe as the participants explored and navigated a virtual town (Ekstrom et al., 2003). The difficulty with these types of recording is that the electrode tip tends to drift away from the neuron as an animal moves but this can be overcome by using special flexible microelectrodes that can shift with the brain. For a more thorough review of the main neuroscience techniques, see Lynch and O'Mara (1997).

Through the combination of these techniques, coupled with clever and innovative experimental designs and incisive research questions, neuroscientists have been able to make significant strides in the past 50 years towards understanding the complex workings of the brain. This book contains a small sample of such work, selected from varying areas within cognitive neuroscience; they encompass vision, memory, plasticity, the motor system, perception, consciousness and attention, employing most of the techniques described above, including neuroimaging (Chapter 7), TMS (Chapters 2 and 8), single/multiple cell recording (Chapter 3), ERPs (Chapters 5 and 6) and behaviour (Chapter 4). It is thanks to studies such as these that we have made such progress in unravelling the mysteries of the human brain.

Note

1   In fact, Golgi asserted this very idea in his Nobel acceptance speech in 1906; he and Cajal had never met previously, and Golgi gave his lecture before Cajal, who would go on to claim the opposite – that nerve cells were discrete entities.

References

Buckner, R. and Logan, J. (2001) Functional neuroimaging methods: PET and fMRI, in R. Cabeza and A. Kingstone (eds) *Handbook of Functional Neuroimaging and Cognition*. Cambridge, MA: MIT Press.

Cacioppo, J.T., Tassinary, L.G. and Berntson, G.G. (2007) *Handbook of Psychophysiology*, 3rd edn. Cambridge: Cambridge University Press.

Ekstrom, A.D., Kahana, M.J., Caplan, J.B., Fields, T.A., Isham, E.A., Newman, E.L. and Fried, I. (2003) Cellular networks underlying human spatial navigation, *Nature*, 425(6954): 184–8.

Hafting, T., Fyhn, M., Bonnevie, T., Moser, M.B. and Moser, E.I. (2008) Hippocampus-independent phase precession in entorhinal grid cells, *Nature*, 453(7199): 1248–52.

Hebb, D.O. (1949) *The Organisation of Behavior*. New York: Wiley.

Hubel, D. and Wiesel, T. (1962) Receptive fields, binocular interaction and functional architecture in the cat's visual cortex, *Journal of Physiology of London*, 160: 106–54.

Kwong, K.K., Belliveau, J.W., Chesler, D.A. et al. (1992) Dynamic magnetic resonance imaging of human brain activity during primary sensory stimulation, *Proceedings of the National Academy of Sciences USA*, 89(12): 5675–9.

Lynch, M.A. and O'Mara, S.M. (1997) (eds) *Neuroscience Labfax*. London: Academic Press.

Murro, A.M., Smith, J.R., King, D.W. and Park, Y.D. (1995) Precision of dipole localization in a spherical volume conductor: a comparison of referential EEG, magnetoencephalography and scalp current density methods, *Brain Topography*, 8(2): 119–25.

Ogawa, S., Lee, T.M., Nayak, A.S. and Glynn, P. (1990) Oxygenation-sensitive contrast in magnetic resonance image of rodent brain at high magnetic fields, *Magnetic Resonance in Medicine*, 14(1): 68–78.

O'Keefe, J. and Dostrovsky, J. (1971) The hippocampus as a spatial map: preliminary evidence from unit activity in the freely-moving rat, *Brain Research*, 34(1): 171–5.

O'Mara, S.M., Rolls, E.T., Berthoz, A. and Kesner, R.P. (1994) Neurons responding to whole-body motion in the primate hippocampus, *Journal of Neuroscience*, 14(11): 6511–23.

Perrett, D.I., Rolls, E.T., Caan, W. (1982) Visual neurones responsive to faces in the monkey temporal cortex, *Experimental Brain Research*, 47(3): 329–42.

Ray, W.J. and Cole, H.W. (1985) EEG activity during cognitive processing: influence of attentional factors, *International Journal of Psychophysiology*, 3(1): 43–8.

Roy, C.S. and Sherrington, C.S. (1890) On the regulation of the blood supply of the brain, *Journal of Physiology*, 11: 85–108.

Taub, E., Miller, N.E., Novack, T.A. et al. (1993) Technique to improve chronic motor deficit after stroke, *Archives of Physical Medicine and Rehabilitation*, 74(4): 347–54.

Taube, J.S., Muller, R.U. and Ranck, J.B. Jr. (1990) Head-direction cells recorded from the postsubiculum in freely moving rats. I. Description and quantitative analysis, *Journal of Neuroscience*, 10(2): 420–35.

2   The malleable brain: neuroplasticity in the motor system

Discussion of:

Pascual-Leone, A., Nguyet, D., Cohen, L.G., Brasil-Neto, J.P., Cammarota, A. and Hallett, M. (1995)

Modulation of muscle responses evoked by transcranial magnetic stimulation during the acquisition of new fine motor skills, *Journal of Neurophysiology*, 74(3): 1037–45

Reprinted with permission from the American Physiological Society © 1995

Foreword, background and description by Richard A.P. Roche and Seán Commins
Author's commentary by Alvaro Pascual-Leone
Peer commentary by Vincent Walsh

Foreword

This chapter discusses a paper that demonstrates quite dramatically the capacity of the human brain to reshape its physical structure as a direct result of repeated experience. The combination of a clever and well-controlled design, the use of a fascinating and appropriate technology and a spectacular set of results ensure its inclusion in this collection of innovative experiments. It shows how repetition of a finger sequence exercise with the right hand, over a five-day period, resulted in expansion of the areas of motor cortex responsible for controlling those fingers. This expansion was larger relative to both a control group who engaged in no finger exercise, and to a group who played piano at will with the right hand for the same length of time. Furthermore, a second study demonstrates how mental practice of the motor sequence resulted in both improvements in performance of the exercise and comparable expansion of motor areas to that seen with actual physical practice.

Introduction

Scientists are often wrong. In fact, the history of scientific endeavour is littered with cases where a belief that was previously held as 'fact' or 'truth' has later been shown to be completely (and sometimes spectacularly) incorrect. The long-held assumption that the earth was flat is probably the best known example, but virtually every field of study has its own embarrassing admission about having got it wrong in the past, and the study of the brain is no exception. Until relatively recently, there existed two widely held beliefs among neuroscientists and physicians alike pertaining to brain structure and neural connectivity. One of these beliefs was that when we are born, our brains contain their full complement of ~10 billion cells, and this collection of neurons could not be added to over time – these were all the cells we would ever have, and their number could not increase, only decrease with cell death through age, damage or disease. Accordingly, advice from medical practitioners with regard to brain injury was stark and pessimistic: 'do not damage your brain, because we cannot replace any cells that you lose'. While it was the received wisdom that our stock of brain cells did not increase over time, it was understood that it was the *connectivity* between these cells that grew and became more elaborate across the lifespan, and that these changes in connectivity seemed to coincide with major advances in cognitive ability; for example, the development of the ability for abstract thought in children. Related to this, the second, long-held belief was that the structure of the mature adult brain was fixed and hard-wired, and that once these developmental growth spurts in connectivity had finished, the structure of the cortex was effectively set in stone. For much of the past century, these two ideas influenced much of the scientific thinking with regard to neural development and brain rehabilitation.

However, in recent decades, both of these beliefs have been shown to be inaccurate. Research has since demonstrated that *neurogenesis*, the creation of new brain cells, is possible under certain conditions and in specific parts of the brain (see Sisken et al., 1990; Ramirez, 1997; Eriksson et al., 1998). In addition, laboratory demonstrations of cell plasticity in various brain regions including the hippocampus (see Bliss and Lomo, 1973, and Chapter 7), visual cortex (Berry et al., 1989; Aroniadou and Teyler, 1992) and somatosensory cortex (Zhang et al., 2000) have shown that physical alterations in cell connectivity as a result of experience are possible in the adult brain. These two factors have proved crucially important for approaches to neurorehabilitation following large-scale cell loss in such cases as stroke; constraint-induced movement therapy, for example, has yielded impressive reports of significant recovery of cognitive function; in some cases even 20 years post-stroke. Other cases that reveal the effects of neuroplasticity at work include recovery of visual attention following left spatial hemineglect (see Chapter 4 for a description of the phenomenon), post-traumatic stress disorder (PTSD) (see Bremner, 1999) and prism adaptation (Frassinetti et al., 2002). Research into neuroplasticity has, therefore, become one of the major fields of inquiry in contemporary neuroscience.

Some of the most dramatic laboratory demonstrations of plasticity were provided by Nudo, Merzenich and colleagues, who carried out a series of studies with monkeys. These studies made use of the fact that the motor cortex of humans and non-human primates alike contains a map of the different parts of the body controlled by that region of cortex (see Figure 2.1). This so-called 'motor homunculus' can be effectively mapped by electrically stimulating a portion of motor cortex and observing which part of the body exhibits movement or twitching. In this way, the cortical areas associated with the control of each of the fingers of the contralateral hand can be outlined.

Merzenich and colleagues carried out exactly this type of cortical mapping at the outset of one of their studies (Nudo et al., 1996), and then created a situation whereby the monkeys were forced to use only the middle and ring fingers of the hand to retrieve

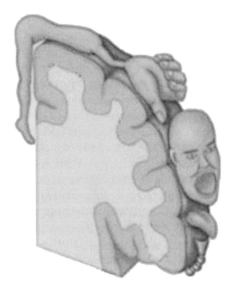 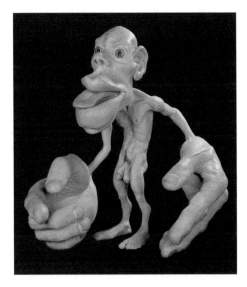

Figure 2.1 Organization of motor cortex and body representations of each portion of cortex (left) and the motor homunculus representing relative cortical extent of each body part by size (right).

Left panel image accessed from: www.brainconnection.com/topics/?main=gal/homunculus
Right panel image accessed from: www.sharpbrains.com/blog/2006/10/04/brain-exercise-who-is-this/

food from a small food-well. After an extended period of this training, the cortical areas associated with the fingers were mapped again, and this mapping revealed expansion of the areas associated with the control of the middle and ring fingers into areas previously devoted to other fingers (see Figure 2.2, page C1). This was a very clear demonstration of use-dependent cortical plasticity and functional cortical expansion. The Pascual-Leone et al. study discussed in this chapter employs a similar methodology applied to human participants, and rather than executing the cortical mapping by electrical stimulation of the cortical surface (necessitating the opening of the skull), the mapping is carried out non-invasively by transcranial magnetic stimulation (TMS). By applying a large and rapidly changing magnetic field to the scalp, cell firing can be induced in the underlying population of neurons, thereby allowing cortical mapping of the motor cortex to be carried out by observing muscle movements and twitches as the TMS coil is placed in different locations on the scalp.

Background and description of the study

Pascual-Leone and colleagues conducted two experiments in which they asked subjects to perform a finger movement exercise on a piano (using just one hand and involving all five digits). All participants had no previous experience of playing the piano or any other musical instrument, nor did they have jobs that involved fine-finger skills. All were right-handed.

In the first experiment, all participants ($n = 18$) had to perform a sequence of finger movements without pauses, fluently and without skipping any key while at the same time trying to keep tempo with a metronome beat. The sequence of fingers and notes used were thumb-C, index finger-D, middle finger-E, ring finger-F, little finger-G, ring finger-F, middle finger-E and index finger-D. On the first day of training the authors divided the participants into three groups. In the first group, participants were initially taught the finger exercise and were then allowed to practise the sequence for two hours each day for five days. Following their daily practice session the participants had their performance tested which, in turn, was followed by TMS mapping of two regions of the motor cortex (representing the finger flexor and extensor muscles). Participants in the second group had daily mapping of the motor cortex by TMS for five days and then on the fifth day were taught the finger exercise followed by a performance test. Participants in the third group were allowed to play the piano at will (anything they wanted) for two hours each day for five days. They were asked not to repeat a given sequence of notes. This was again followed each day by TMS mapping. On the fifth day, the third group was taught the finger exercise, which was then followed by a performance test.

Results showed that the playing skills of the first group improved greatly over the five days, with their error rates in the sequence of key presses decreasing daily. Figure 2.3 (top) shows this decrease in errors and Figure 2.3 (bottom) compares the performance of one individual on the first day compared to that of the fifth. As would be expected the error rates for the second and third groups were very high given that these were only taught the exercise on day five and then given the performance test immediately.

Importantly, when the TMS cortical output maps for the three groups were compared, the authors found that there was a significant and gradual increase in the cortical motor areas representing the finger flexor and extensor muscles for the trained group (Group 1) across the five days of training (Figure 2.4 top). Interestingly, although the cortical representation size for Group 3 (the group that was allowed to randomly play each day) had also increased over the five days, the increase was significantly smaller than that of the practised group (see Figure 2.4 bottom). As would be expected, there were no changes in the cortical representation of the group that underwent TMS mapping only (Group 2).

In a second experiment, the authors randomly assigned 15 participants to three groups. All subjects were taught the same five-finger exercise as in Experiment 1 and all had TMS mapping of the motor cortical areas representing the long finger flexor and extensor muscles. The first group (physical practice group), similar to Experiment 1, were requested to practise on the piano keyboard for two hours each day for five days. Following each daily practice session they were tested on their performance and this was followed up 20–30 minutes later by the TMS mapping session. The second group (mental practice group) was requested to sit at a piano and try to visualize their fingers performing the exercise and to imagine the sound. They were requested not to move their fingers or touch the piano. This mental practice also took place two hours daily for five days, followed by a daily performance test and TMS mapping. On the fifth day participants in this group were allowed to mentally practise, followed by a performance test and a mapping session; they were then allowed to practise the exercise physically for a further two hours that was again followed by a performance

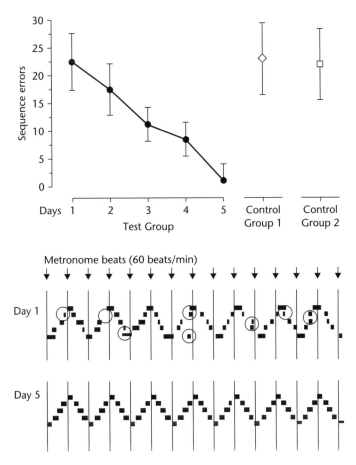

Figure 2.3 (Top) Interval between key presses and number of sequence errors for all over the course of five days' learning. (Bottom) A representative test subject on days 1 and 5. Arrows and dashed lines mark the metronome beats. Bars illustrate the different notes. Circles highlight the errors in the sequence performance.

Source: Reprinted with permission from the American Physiological Society: *Journal of Neurophysiology* (Pascual-Leone et al., 1995), © (1995).

test. The third group (control) was only given a daily performance test followed by a TMS mapping session. This group was not allowed to practise the exercise physically or mentally.

Results from this experiment demonstrated that the physical practice group improved significantly over the five days, with their error rates in the sequence of key presses decreasing daily (Figure 2.5, closed circles). In addition, the mental practice group did improve slightly over the five days but they were significantly worse than the physical practice group by day five (Figure 2.5, open circle day five). In fact, their performance was comparable to day three of the physical practice group (black arrows). However, with the extra two hours of physical exercise on the fifth day, the performance of the mental practice group improved significantly and was by then equivalent to the

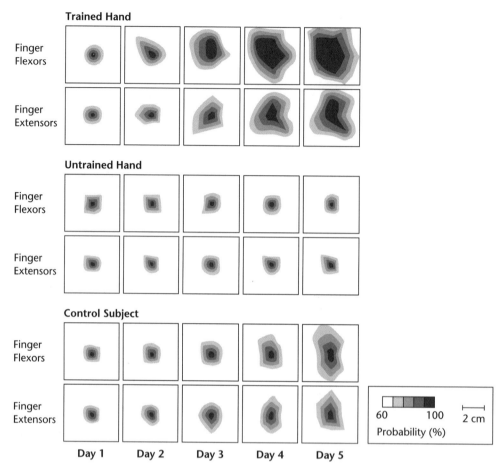

Figure 2.4 Representative examples of the cortical motor output maps for the long finger flexor and extensor muscles on days 1–5 in a test subject (trained and untrained hand) and a subject from control group 2.

Source: Reprinted with permission from the American Physiological Society: *Journal of Neurophysiology* (Pascual-Leone et al., 1995), © (1995).

physical exercise group (Figure 2.5, stippled grey circle day 5). As would be expected, the control group's performance remained poor throughout the week (Figure 2.5, grey squares).

Interestingly, results from the TMS mapping sessions indicated that the size of the motor areas representing the finger flexors and the finger extensions increased daily in both the physical practice group *and* the mental exercise group (Figure 2.6, top and middle panels), while the size of the cortical output map did not change for the control group (Figure 2.6, bottom panel). However, despite the poorer performance of the mental practice group compared to the physical practice group (particularly by day five, see Figure 2.5), plastic changes were occurring in the motor cortex of the mental practice group that were equivalent to those in the physical practice group.

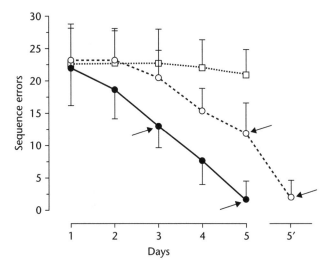

Figure 2.5 Number of sequence errors for all over the course of 5 days' learning. (Filled circles = physical practice group; open circles = mental practice group; stippled squares = control group; stippled circle = mental practice group on day 5).

Source: Reprinted with permission from the American Physiological Society: *Journal of Neurophysiology* (Pascual-Leone et al., 1995), © (1995).

This study reveals a number of important implications for plasticity in the motor system of the human brain. Primarily, the data clearly show that physical practice of a motor sequence results in a behavioural enhancement of performance, which is mirrored by an expansion of the extent of cortical tissue devoted to the control of the specific area concerned. This gives a significant insight into the structural brain changes that take place as a direct consequence of repeated physical activity, and this may prove particularly pertinent for athletes, musicians and indeed any person who engages in repetitive execution of a directed set of motor commands. In fact, the recent prevalence of text communication via a mobile phone has most likely led to cortical expansion of regions governing the thumb of many mobile users. Furthermore, the finding that imagined practice can lead to some performance gains and comparable cortical expansion is a point that has become highly significant in the area of sports psychology. Many sports psychologists now emphasize the importance of mental rehearsal of the desired motor action (e.g. serving in tennis, shooting in basketball/football, stroke execution in golf), but the findings of Pascual-Leone et al. strongly suggest that such visualization techniques are most effective when accompanied by even a minimal amount of physical practice. Finally, the results offer an optimistic outlook for many realms within neurorehabilitation including disorders that involve large-scale loss of neurons such as stroke, PTSD and Alzheimer's disease. This demonstration of neural plasticity and cortical reorganization implies that, through repeated mental and/or physical exercise, the remaining brain tissue has the capacity to re-establish functioning circuits by means of the growth of new connections, even after serious damage and cell loss.

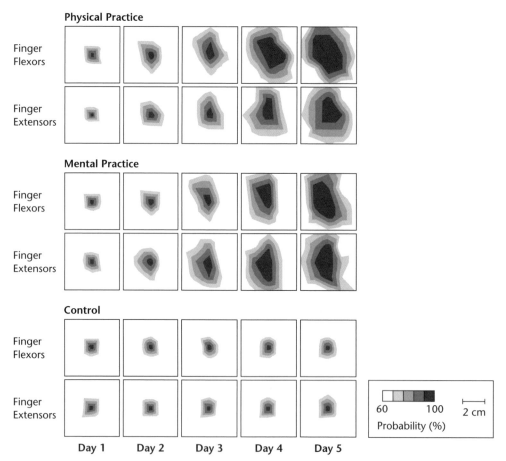

Figure 2.6 Representative examples of the cortical motor output maps for the long finger flexor and extensor muscles on days 1–5 in a subject from each group in Experiment 2.

Source: Reprinted with permission from the American Physiological Society: *Journal of Neurophysiology* (Pascual-Leone et al., 1995), © (1995).

Author commentary by Alvaro Pascual-Leone

In 'The Last Lecture', Randy Pausch's moving message to his children and life advice to all, stresses the importance of childhood dreams: pursuing one's own and enabling the dreams of others. This does seem like sound advice to me, and I was fortunate, after quite a bit of back and forth, to finally figure out that I wanted to study how the human brain enabled us to learn new skills, to create, to become self-aware, to imagine the future. I presume that most of us in cognitive neuroscience have a similar story and motivation. In my case my parents, both physicians, and my uncle, a psychologist who trained initially as a physician and became a psychiatrist before studying with Piaget, strongly encouraged me to go to medical school and become a neurologist in order to pursue these goals. I had thought of studying philosophy, mathematics and psychology, but eventually I did follow their advice and went to medical school and became a neurologist. Of course, once you formulate a dream, and embrace it, and devote yourself to achieving it, you are changed by the endeavor, and eventually become unable to even fathom why you ever had doubts as to what dreams to pursue. The Spanish philosopher Ortega-y-Gasset pointed out that, when confronted with a really important decision in life, the only critical requirement is to actually decide. What the decision might be is less important, since, as he put it, if you make a decision and commit yourself to it, you will be changed by the decision, and thus, you shall never be able to regret it. So, childhood dreams and their committed pursuit are important, and I was fortunate to have those.

In addition to dreams, you need good mentors. I attended medical school at the Albert-Ludwigs University in Freiburg (Germany) where I completed an MD/PhD programme, writing my thesis on the neurophysiology of proprioceptive inputs into the vestibular nuclei of the cat. Professor Richard Jung was at the end of his career, already afflicted by the deficits of a stroke, but he remained an impressive influence to a young, enthusiastic student. Richard was full of life, curiosity, precise thinking, extensive knowledge of the work of others, careful experimentation and never-ending encouragement to beginners. After completing my MD/PhD programme in Freiburg I went to the USA and received my neurology training at the University of Minnesota where I also completed a fellowship in clinical neurophysiology. In Minnesota I was fortunate to meet Professor David Anderson, currently the Chairman of Neurology at the University of Minnesota, then at Hennepin County Medical Center. David is a superb clinician and teacher who was critical in my training as a neurologist. He also encouraged me to pursue my interest in research and I began to work on direct cortical stimulation and TMS at the Minnesota Comprehensive Epilepsy Program. TMS had only recently been introduced by Anthony Barker in 1985 and I was able to work on the development of the first repetitive magnetic stimulation device; I received from John Cadwell the first repetitive magnetic stimulator prototype and began a series of studies on the use of TMS in epilepsy and in language mapping.

In 1991 I joined Mark Hallett at the Human Motor Control Section at the National Institute of Neurological Disorders and Stroke (Bethesda, Maryland) for a fellowship in human cortical physiology and human motor control. This fellowship offered me the opportunity to continue the work with TMS and gain experience in movement disorders, motor control and human-based research. Once again, I was extremely fortunate to find an outstanding mentor in Mark Hallett. The four years I spent at the National Institute of Health (NIH) crystallized my resolve to devote myself to the study of systems physiology and human cortical physiology with the aim of understanding brain plasticity and guiding it with neurophysiologic techniques. The present experiment dates back to that time and is one of a series on the modulation of motor cortical outputs during the acquisition of new skills. This work was critical in shaping my thinking about the possible application of neuromodulation to study and guide neuroplasticity, and the potential of TMS as a non-invasive method to test such principles. In shaping these ideas, my mentor, Mark, was very influential, always willing to listen and discuss concepts, aptly combining advice, guidance and freedom for me to pursue my own thoughts. If a mentor can be defined as an active partner in an ongoing relationship who helps a mentee maximize potential and reach personal and professional goals, then Mark was the perfect mentor for me, and I find myself trying to emulate him in my own mentoring efforts.

At Mark's laboratory I was keen on studying how the brain changes in the setting of the acquisition of new skills. Jordan Grafman was using the serial reaction time task (SRTT) in some studies on procedural learning in various patient populations. I learned about the task, used it in some experiments on patients with Parkinson's disease and cerebellar lesions, and reached to the conclusion that the SRTT might offer an ideal test to explore the modulation of motor cortical outputs during implicit procedural learning and the eventual transition to explicit knowledge. I had subjects perform blocks of the SRTT and obtained their motor output maps serially after each block of the task. The findings were remarkable, revealing a progressive enlargement of the motor cortical output maps during the implicit learning and a rather sudden change, with return to a smaller output maps when the subjects became explicitly aware of the sequence being learned in the SRTT. This gave rise to a paper in *Science* (Pascual-Leone et al., 1994) and I was eager to pursue related experiments.

Fortunately, Hunter Fry from Australia spent some time at Mark's laboratory, and he and they set up a MIDI keyboard to study motor coordination in pianists with and without overuse syndrome. Mark was interested in this line of work as it might relate to focal, task-specific dystonia. Hunter Fry is an expert in the painful musculoligamentous overuse in the arms and hands of pianists (overuse syndrome) and wanted to quantify its impact on motor control. They were studying pianists with overuse syndrome and skill-matched pianists with no history of overuse. The pianists were asked to perform continuous repetitions of a five-finger exercise on a piano keyboard at metronome-paced tempos. The main outcome measures were quantitative analysis of four measurements of performance (duration of key presses, interval between key presses, velocity of key presses and time off the metronome beat). Nguyet Dang, a very gifted research technician, had helped set up the equipment and write the necessary programs to be able to obtain the desired information from the MIDI keyboard.

Around that time I had read Santiago Ramón y Cajal's thoughts on brain plasticity in his 1904 *Textura del Sistema Nervioso* in which he wrote that:

> The labor of a pianist [. . .] is inaccessible for the uneducated man as the acquisition of new skill requires many years of mental and physical practice. In order to fully understand this complex phenomenon it becomes necessary to admit, in addition to the reinforcement of pre-established organic pathways, the formation of new pathways through ramification and progressive growth of the dendritic arborization and the nervous terminals.
>
> (Ramón y Cajal 1904)

Thus, I wondered whether I might be able to use the MIDI keyboard and the programmed measures to examine the changes in motor cortical output induced by the physical and mental practice required to learn a five-finger movement exercise in untrained participants. Mark was supportive of the idea and with the help of Nguyet, Leonardo Cohen, Joaquim Brasil-Neto and Angel Cammarota we set out to run the experiment. Having participants practice a five-finger movement exercise on a piano keyboard for two hours per day, daily for a week, is hard. We spent many hours in a small laboratory encouraging subjects to concentrate and focus. During the mental practice version of the experiment we had to contain our anxiety at not knowing what the subjects were actually doing while sitting in front of the keyboard, resting their fingers on the keys after having been instructed to rehearse mentally. The execution of the experiment was rather tedious, but the results were exciting, and with each new participant our enthusiasm grew.

Thus, it is noteworthy that in addition to dreams and mentors, serendipity is also important, and you must be willing and able to embrace it. Horace Walpole coined the word serendipity in 1754 in a letter to a friend, derived from the fairy tale *The Three Princes of Serendip*. He wrote: 'as their highnesses traveled, they were always making discoveries, by accidents and sagacity, of things which they were not in quest of' and referred to it as 'accidental sagacity (for you must observe that no discovery of a thing you are looking for, comes under this description)'. Thus, serendipity is not just luck or a chance encounter, but requires 'sagacity', the ability to make the link between apparently innocuous facts and thus reach a valuable conclusion. The concept is reminiscent of Louis Pasteur's famous sentence: 'In the fields of observation chance favors only the prepared mind'.

Peer commentary by Vincent Walsh

When I agreed to write this peer commentary I did so without knowing which one of Alvaro Pascual-Leone's many landmark papers the editors would select for special attention. Their choice of the 1995 learning paper is a good one: the paper is important for many reasons and it is representative of (perhaps it was even the beginning of) what in my own view is Alvaro's most important contribution to date – his challenge to the idea that the sensory cortex is, well, 'merely' sensory and that sensory specializations are cast in stone (e.g. Pascual-Leone et al., 2005). It follows from this approach that the limits of plasticity in the brain are also open to question and the paper discussed in this book opens a valuable avenue of research and continues to inspire new ideas and experiments. The value of the paper has three components: the link between thought and action; plasticity; and prospects for rehabilitation.

The link between thought and action is one that is given much lip service but here it is tested and limits are set. The basic finding that the area of scalp from which the motor cortex could be stimulated increased following training was a beautiful demonstration in itself, but the hook is that a similar change occurs when people imagine the same task. Thinking *is* doing, after all. I have heard some musicians claim that merely thinking about a new piece of music is the equivalent of physically practising and we are now familiar with athletes mentally practising their events. The important question is *what are the limits of mental practice?* In the 1995 paper, the increase in motor cortex sensitivity following motor practice was similar to that following real practice. Why was this? To answer this I need to turn to one of Alvaro's unpublished observations; the fact that over several summers when I visited his house in New England I would beat him at one-on-one basketball in his driveway. We played often and I am sure Alvaro *thought* about beating me but the first limit on plasticity and mental practice is that mental practice and fantasy are not the same thing. The gains from mental practice require that you *can* perform the actions and therefore be able to activate the same neural assemblies as used during the real thing. The same message is strengthened by the lack of changes in motor sensitivity in the control group who made piano key presses at will: as well as the imagined act being possible, it is necessary for the act being practised to be organized. This simple fact is a hard one to teach people: half an hour of 'good' (i.e. organized and goal-directed) practice, 'good' (i.e. concentrated and thoughtful) reading or 'good' (i.e. intense and good technical) exercise is always better than the three hours of the desperate catch-up that we have all done out of fear of the upcoming exam or the guilt of holiday excesses.

One of the questions less often addressed in discussions of plasticity is the price of plasticity and we can look to this study as a guide for where to start. Although the TMS measures show similar changes at a global level (Figure 2.4), the behavioural outcome for mental practice is not as great as for real practice (Figure 2.5). This may be a simple function of stronger associations and feedback in the physical practice condition but it raises the deeper issue of the price of plasticity. Common examples of 'bad' plasticity are musicians' dystonia and writer's cramp wherein the over-representation or fusion of highly trained muscle representations cause a loss of ability. This means that when we take learning paradigms outside the laboratory into the rehab clinic, the school academy or the music conservatoire, we have to be aware that plasticity has limits and that those limits may be reached more readily in damaged or developing brains. The right kind of practice includes the right kind of rest. Teachers and physiotherapists may be forgiven for thinking that neuroscientists are reinventing the wheel here but they would be mistaken. The behavioural heuristics developed for education and rehabilitation will themselves benefit from understanding the physiological basis and limits of plasticity.

This study has been a direct inspiration to hundreds of scientists studying plasticity and I was one of the many who followed it with a related question. In the Pascual-Leone et al. study we see the physiological expression of mental and physical practice, but the brain can respond in more ways than recruiting more neurons and increasing sensitivity. Indeed the opposite can happen – learning can result in greater efficiency and thus in fewer neurons being used for a task. Practice can also result in an area required for learning not being involved when the subject acquires expertise.

In between basketball lessons Alvaro and I spent some time writing a book together; our discussion of the experiments of the 1995 paper is central to a chapter entitled 'The Self-Engineering Brain'. In that chapter we address why thinking might be so effective at inducing motor plasticity and we articulated a position we believe that psychologists, physiologists and cognitive neuroscientists still need to confront. It is the fact that plasticity is not something imposed on or exercised by the brain as an occasional response to new demands – plasticity is the baseline state of the brain; it is ever-changing; ever-consolidating; always making new connections; always making new false memories; and always forgetting. It is this normal state of plasticity that underlies our abilities to learn and relearn skills as we get older and it is one of the hopes for the future of rehabilitation that we will be able to harness this normal ability of plasticity.

The paper presented in this book underpins subsequent and future progress because it took a 'well-understood' area (the motor cortex), simple tasks, a brave hypothesis and provided simple, highly replicable results that have deep implications for the way we conceptualize cortical plasticity. The experiment was, to use the term deservingly for once, 'elegant'.

So where next? Well one option is to take a brainless view of the consequences of this paper and subsequent findings. We can make companies rich by buying 'brain training' consoles but if this isn't bad plasticity, it is an example of pointless plasticity. What needs to be made clear to people is that you tend to get better at the things you practise – generalization of learning is much rarer and difficult to engineer (if Alvaro wants to beat me at basketball it will do him no good to practice soccer). We can also abuse the findings in celebrity books that will teach us how to 'think yourself thin'. But we can also do better and ask how the brain constantly remodels itself, and the 1995 paper is a great starting point. It was no surprise to me that in his commentary Alvaro cited Ramón y Cajal. I know that Alvaro's approach to plasticity and science in general is inspired by a love of the history of his subject and also the appreciation that knowing the history of exploration of your subject is an obligation not an indulgence. In writing the 'Self-Engineering' chapter together we concluded that 'Plasticity is not a special state of the nervous system – *plasticity is the normal state of the nervous system*'. This simple fact is a hard one for many experimenters to accept (damn it, it makes experiments harder) but it is only one of many such difficulties we have to face in understanding the brain. From here we have a base from which to face other difficulties such as the limits of sensory, modularity, reorganization following injury, education and how to beat your friends at basketball: imagine that.

References

Aroniadou, V.A. and Teyler, T.J. (1992) Induction of NMDA receptor independent long-term potentiation (LTP) in visual cortex of adult rats, *Brain Research*, 584: 169–73.

Berry, R.L., Teyler, T.J. and Taizhen, H. (1989) Induction of LTP in rat primary visual cortex: tetanus parameters, *Brain Research*, 481: 221–7.

Bliss, T.V. and Lomo, T. (1973) Long-lasting potentiation of synaptic transmission in the dentate area of the anaesthetized rabbit following stimulation of the perforant path, *Journal of Physiology*, 232: 331–56.

Bremner, J.D. (1999) Does stress damage the brain? *Biological Psychiatry*, 45: 797–805.

Eriksson, P.S., Perfilieva, E., Björk-Eriksson, T., Alborn, A.M., Nordborg, C., Peterson, D.A. and Gage, F.H. (1998) Neurogenesis in the adult human hippocampus, *Nature Medicine*, 4: 1313–17.

Frassinetti, F., Angeli, V., Meneghello, F., Avanzi, S. and Làdavas, E. (2002) Long-lasting amelioration of visuospatial neglect by prism adaptation, *Brain*, 125(3): 608–23.

Nudo, R.J., Milliken, G.W., Jenkins, W.M. and Merzenich, M.M. (1996) Use-dependent alterations of movement representations in primary motor cortex of adult squirrel monkeys, *Journal of Neuroscience*, 16(2): 785–807.

Pascual-Leone, A., Amedi, A., Fregni, F. and Merabet, L.B. (2005) The plastic human brain cortex, *Annual Review of Neuroscience*, 28: 377–401.

Pascual-Leone, A., Grafman, J. and Hallett, M. (1994) Modulation of cortical motor output maps during development of implicit and explicit knowledge, *Science*, 263(5151): 1287–9.

Ramirez, J.J. (1997) The functional significance of lesion-induced plasticity of the hippocampal formation in H.J. Freund, B.A. Sabel and O.W. Witte (eds), *Brain Plasticity: Advances in Neurology*, pp. 61–78. Philadelphia, PA: Lippencott-Raven Publishers.

Ramón y Cajal, S. (1904) *La Textura del Sistema Nerviosa del Hombre y los Vertebrados*. Madrid: Moya.

Sisken, B.F., Kanje, M., Lundborg, G. and Kurtz, W. (1990) Pulsed electromagnetic fields stimulate nerve regeneration in vitro and in vivo, *Restorative Neurological Neuroscience*, 1: 303–9.

Zhang, Z., Nguyen, K. and Krnjevic, K. (2000) 2-deoxyglucose induces LTP in layer I of rat somatosensory cortex in vitro, *Brain Research*, 876: 103–11.

3   Monkey see, monkey do: frontal lobe cells that mimic observed actions

Discussion of:

Rizzolatti, G., Fadiga, L., Gallese, V. and Fogassi, L. (1996)

Premotor cortex and the recognition of motor actions, *Cognitive Brain Research*, 3(2): 131–41

Reprinted with permission from Elsevier © 1996

Foreword, background and description by Richard A.P. Roche and Seán Commins
Author's commentary by Luciano Fadiga
Peer commentary by V.S. Ramachandran

Foreword

While much of neuroscience and neuropsychology is concerned with the way large regions of brain tissue – lobes, sub-regions, specific sulci or gyri – function and contribute to behaviour, the properties of individual groups of neurons can prove equally revealing about aspects of processing. In this chapter, we look at some experiments that investigate the remarkable firing properties of a sub-group of frontal cortical cells in monkeys, which have become known as 'mirror neurons', and which may provide important insights into such capacities as vicarious learning, communication and possibly speech production. The subsequent finding of an apparently comparable system in humans makes the significance of these cells all the greater.

Introduction

Neurons are quite remarkable cells. Though vast in number, with tens of billions packed into every human brain, they can be classified based on structure into a handful of broad categories. They are diverse in function, too; some act as carriers of information, others hold these signallers in place and further ones roam about, gobbling up waste. Their activity is controlled largely by the comings and goings of charged particles into and out of the membrane, with voltage-controlled ion channels dictating whether a signal passed down from another cell will be shunted onwards to its neighbour, or suppressed, breaking the chain of communication. They grow and sprout new connections as long as they are fed with new experience, reaching out towards nearby cells that happen to fire at the same time. Such acquaintances last a long time, and may form the basis for memories that endure for a lifetime.

But perhaps most remarkable feature of neurons is the range and diversity of events that will cause them to fire, to pass on their message to their neighbours. Some will respond to sounds, others to visual inputs, yet more to imagined experiences. Some are selective for places, some for movements, others for memories of events. Early sensory neurons are some of the easiest to entice into firing – simple line segments will suffice for early V1 visual cells, while crude phonemes will activate their early auditory counterparts. As one travels upstream in the cortex, the cells are more difficult to please. Higher-order visual cells in ventral temporal areas will only deign to fire in response to faces, others to specific classes of objects. And as we move higher still into multisensory areas, we encounter cells capable of responding to stimulation from more than one type of input. Such idiosyncrasies in firing preference have fascinated neuroscientists for decades, and research using single- or multiple-cell recording techniques in non-human primates has led to some truly amazing revelations about the nature of such cells, while also giving clues to the workings of the larger circuits within which they operate.

Among the most fascinating single-unit studies of recent years are those of Giacomo Rizzolatti and colleagues, who investigated a sub-population of neurons in the frontal area F5 of the monkey. These neurons showed the remarkable characteristic of firing in response to a particular observed movement by the experimenter, *and* in response to a comparable movement by the monkey. In some cases, the experimenter (or, in subsequent studies, another monkey) would manipulate a piece of food, causing these 'mirror cells' to fire furiously. Firing would then cease until the monkey engaged in a similar motor activity itself, with this movement accompanied by another major burst of cell firing. Various careful control conditions were used to rule out the possibility that these cells were activating in preparation to make a movement; for example to take a piece of food. It appeared that these cells formed part of a specific observation/ execution network, one that receives massive input from area AIP in inferior parietal lobule, a region known to be involved in hand movements and different types of hand grip for interacting with objects. Further, random hand movements were insufficient to elicit the pattern of mirrored firing; rather, the gestures must have some *meaning* for the animal, some functional significance, in order to produce this reciprocated activation. Rizzolatti and colleagues speculated that when the animal observed an action, which was already in its own behavioural repertoire of stored movement sequences, the system would automatically make that movement sequence available to the animal, in case rapid reciprocation of the movement was required.

In addition, Rizzolatti and co-workers subsequently obtained data from a magnetic stimulation study suggesting strongly that a comparable system exists in the human brain. But what could the possible utility of such a system be for humans, aside from the ability to mimic the movements of another? A clue may come from the neuroanatomy of the region in which the mirror cells were found. Area F5 is part of the agranular frontal cortex of the monkey, and appears to have a dorsal–ventral division of function: cells in the dorsal region appear to represent hand movements, while ventral cells are responsible for (and responsive to) movements of the mouth. Most significantly, this region in the monkey is thought to be a possible homologue of Broca's area in the human brain, the frontal speech production area that takes its name from Paul Broca's case study of his aphasic patient Tan (Broca, 1865). The authors suggest that the observed firing of the mirror cells in F5 may indicate the role of this area in a rudimentary communication system from our evolutionary past, one that was reliant on hand and facial gestures. With the development of language in humans, the region's function may have changed to primarily subserve speech production, with an associated growth of the mouth-movement ventral region at the expense of the hand-related dorsal part of F5, leading to the development of what we know today as Broca's area. As such, studying the behaviour of these mirror cells may tell us more than simply how we can imitate what we see; rather, they may provide insights into the evolution of spoken language in the human race.

Background and description of the study

Rizzolatti et al. recorded single neurons from two monkeys (*Macaca nemestrina*) using tungsten microelectrodes. Recordings were made from area F5 of the frontal cortex. Area F5 is considered homologous to Broca's area in the human brain and is located just behind the lower arm of the arcuate sulcus (see Figure 3.1, shaded area). Previous stimulation and recording experiments have shown that this area is related to both hand and mouth movements, with hand movements associated with the dorsal part of area F5 and mouth movements with the more ventral parts of this structure (Rizzolatti et al., 1988).

Initially, all neurons recorded from area F5 were tested for various behavioural capacities, including reactivity to objects and grasping properties. Typically, items of various sizes and shapes were presented in a test box that was placed in front of the

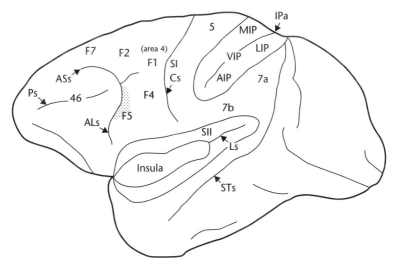

Figure 3.1 Lateral view of the monkey brain. The shaded area shows the anatomical localization of the recorded neurons.

Source: Reprinted with permission from Elsevier: *Cognitive Brain Research* (Rizzolatti et al., 1996), © (1996).

monkey; the monkey was required initially to press a switch that illuminated the box containing the objects. This was then followed by a short delay (1.5 seconds maximum), after which the box's door opened and the monkey was allowed to grasp the object. In addition, F5 neurons' responses were also tested for various motor actions performed in front of the monkey. These actions included presentation of food, putting the food in front of the monkey, taking the food away or giving the food to a second person. Other food-related motor actions included breaking or tearing the food. Finally, a set of non-food/object-related actions were also performed in front of the monkey; these included lifting arms and waving hands. All actions were performed to the animal's left and right, repeated several times and at various distances from the monkey.

Of the 300 neurons recorded from area F5, 20 per cent were classified as 'mirror neurons', defined as those neurons that became responsive when the monkey observed *meaningful hand actions* performed by the experimenter. These neurons did not simply respond to objects (whether presented in isolation or by hand), nor did they simply respond to the motor action itself (grasping, reaching, etc.). Rather, there had to be some interaction between the movement and the object that would carry some *meaning* for the animal, such as the picking up of food. For example, about 60 per cent of the neurons responded to grasping, with some responding to the grasping action by the monkey and others responded to the grasping action of both the experimenter and the monkey. The majority of the neurons responded to the grasping actions by the monkey. Figure 3.2 shows the experimenter grasping a piece of food

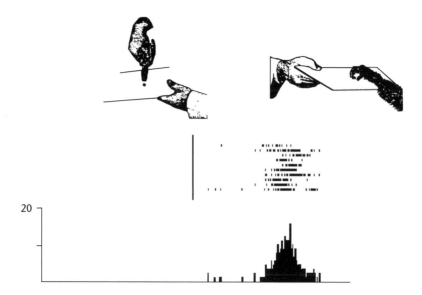

Figure 3.2 Visual and motor responses of a mirror neuron. The behavioral situation is schematically represented in the upper part of the panel. The lower part shows a series of consecutive rasters and the relative peristimulus response histogram. Here, the experimenter grasps the food with a tool. The neuron discharges during grasping observation, ceases to fire when the food is moved and discharges again when the monkey grasps it.

Source: Reprinted with permission from Elsevier: *Cognitive Brain Research* (Rizzolatti et al., 1996), © (1996).

from a tray with a tool; the tray is then moved towards the monkey, and the monkey in turn grasps the piece of food. In this case the neuron only fires as a result of the monkey's own grasping action, and not during the observed grasping of food by the experimenter or the movement of the tray. The absence of neuronal discharge before the monkey's grasping action rules out the possibility that these neurons are 'motor preparation neurons'. Motor preparation neurons, often seen in the pre-motor supplementary area, discharge immediately before a given motor action and are thought to involve the selection of movements that need to be executed.

However, the response of neurons to the grasping action of both the experimenter and the monkey is typical of the mirror neurons, and Figure 3.3 gives an illustrative example of this. Initially, the monkey observes the experimenter grasping a piece of food from a tray; the tray is then moved toward the monkey, and the monkey in turn grasps the food piece. The recorded neuron responds to the experimenter grasping the food, stops firing as the tray is moved towards the monkey and then resumes firing as the monkey grasps the food.

In addition, some mirror neurons discharge as a result of very specific observed actions. Figure 3.4A shows a neuron responding to the observed rotational movement executed by the experimenter's hands around a small piece of food. The neuron responds specifically to anticlockwise rotations. The same neuron responds again

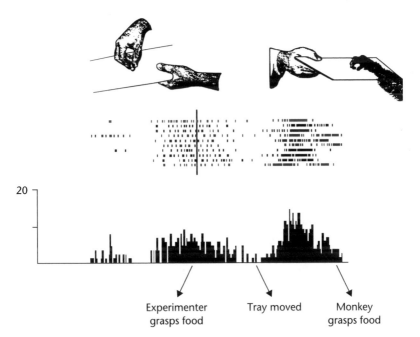

Figure 3.3 The experimenter grasps a piece of food with his hand and moves it towards the monkey who, at the end of the trial, grasps it. The neuron discharges during grasping observation, ceases to fire when the food is moved and discharges again when the monkey grasps it.

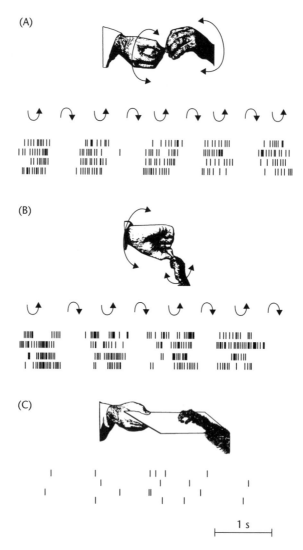

Figure 3.4 Example of a highly congruent mirror neuron. (A) The monkey observes the experimenter who rotates his hands around a raisin in opposite directions alternating clockwise and counterclockwise movements. The response is present only in one rotation direction. (B) The experimenter rotates a piece of food held by the monkey who opposes the experimenter movement making a wrist rotation movement in the opposite direction. (C) Monkey grasps food using a precision grip. Four continuous recordings are shown in each panel. Small arrows above the records indicate the direction of rotations.

Source: Reprinted with permission from Elsevier: *Cognitive Brain Research* (Rizzolatti et al., 1996), © (1996).

when the monkey performs a similar anticlockwise rotational action as he takes the food from the experimenter (Figure 3.4B). There is no neural response when the monkey grasps the food from the tray (Figure 3.4C).

Finally, to rule out the possibility that the responses of these neurons were due to some unintentional interactions between the monkey and the experimenter, a second monkey was used. In this experiment, mirror neurons were recorded from monkey A, while monkey B performed the actions. Figure 3.5 shows that there is a discharge of neural firing from monkey A as it observes the experimenter grasping a piece of food from a tray (Figure 3.5B). There is also a neural response from monkey A if the second monkey grasps the food (Figure 3.5A). In addition, if monkey A grasps the food itself, there is again a neural response from the mirror neuron (Figure 3.5C).

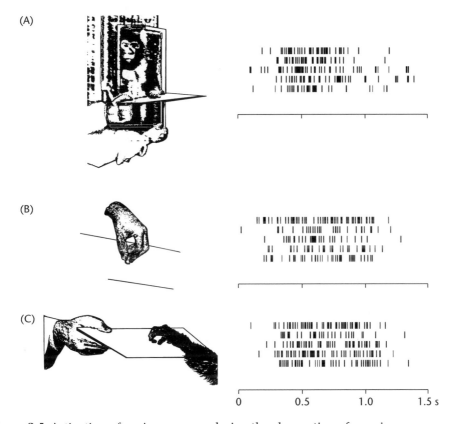

Figure 3.5 Activation of a mirror neuron during the observation of grasping movements performed by a monkey seated in front of the recorded monkey (A), by the experimenter (B) and during the execution of grasping performed by the recorded monkey (C). Each panel illustrates five records of 1.5 s. The spontaneous activity was virtually absent. The neuron discharge was triggered either by the observation or execution of grasping movements.

Source: Reprinted with permission from Elsevier: *Cognitive Brain Research* (Rizzolatti et al., 1996), © (1996).

Author commentary by Luciano Fadiga

The story behind this paper is one of enthusiasm, friendship and serendipity, but more importantly, the outcome of doing research in an exceptional environment.

I started my scientific career in 1985, studying sleep in rats at the University of Bologna, where I worked as an intern for the last two years of medical school. For as long as I can remember, I have never fostered any doubts that I would pursue a career in research, a career I have been fortunate enough to achieve. However, later, after leaving Bologna for Parma to attain my PhD in neuroscience, I realized that there are at least two categories of people in science. The 'reductionists', who think that knowledge *per se* is limited because it deals with infinite problems, and the 'optimists', who think that it is not a crime to pose broad questions like 'how does the brain act on the external world?'. I deeply respect people in both categories. Moreover, I think that a reductionist approach provides young researchers with sound methods and discipline, and it makes the tedious daily work tolerable. When I arrived in Parma and I spoke for the first time with Giacomo Rizzolatti, I remember going back home in the evening telling myself: 'So, it *is* possible to undertake the kind of research I always hoped for . . . !'.

The first study I was involved in sought to formally investigate the behaviour of some strange pre-motor neurons lying in the caudal part of ventral area 6 (area F4), which were responding when the monkey was making proximal movements of the arm, neck, trunk and leg. I say 'strange neurons' because, in addition to these motor properties, many of them also had tactile receptive fields and, more interestingly, they responded to tactile stimulation *before the stimulus even touched the skin*! A visual response in a motor neuron? We discovered that these peripersonal visual receptive fields were anchored onto the tactile ones, meaning that they were not simply driven by eye movement. This meant that the coordinate system characterizing the visual system had been transformed by the brain in a coordinate system centered on body parts. This work led to several publications, including the science paper we wrote (Rizzolatti et al., 1997) to comment on similar findings by Gross and Graziano (Graziano et al., 1997).

It may seem that the F4 neurons described above have nothing to do with the mirror neurons of the brain paper on which I am supposed to comment here. It may seem like mirror neurons miraculously 'popped out' while we were looking for something else and that those of us who were in the lab have benefited from this miracle of serendipity. This is what some people say because it makes an appealing story; particularly for a large audience! But this is not true. Mirror neurons are conceptually like the F4 neurons mapping the peripersonal space in motor coordinates. They map others' actions onto our own motor repertoire. I discuss this point further later in this commentary. Before doing that, I will say a few words about the true story of their discovery.

In 1990 or 1991 (I would definitely have to check the lab protocols), Giuseppe di Pellegrino, Leonardo Fogassi, Vittorio Gallese and I were recording single neurons in monkey area F5, located just in front of area F4. The general aim of the study was to explore the behaviour of other strange neurons (in Parma we were always studying strange things . . . !), originally described by Rizzolatti and co-workers in 1988. These 'strange' neurons, which comprise 20 per cent of F5 neurons, discharged not only during hand grasping (motor response), as is the case in the remaining 80 per cent, but they also discharged when the monkey observed a graspable *object*, compatible (in size and shape) with the *type* of grasping coded by a specific neuron. In other words, if one of these neurons responds to the observation of a small object like a raisin (but not to, say, a banana), it also motorically codes the type of pinch grip required to grasp the raisin. We consequently called these neurons 'canonical neurons' (Rizzolatti and Fadiga, 1998) because they were the F5 visuo-motor neurons doing the job they were expected to do.

During the period when we were working on these experiments in area F5, we all used to have a quick lunch in the lab. Thus, the monkey remained seated on the chair looking at us for about half an hour. I remember that during one of these frugal lunches, simultaneously with the biting of a sandwich, we clearly heard the discharge of a neuron through the loudspeaker connected to the amplifier. The true identity of the biter remains a mystery to this day. Neither can anyone say whether it was really a sandwich or perhaps an ice cream! This is, however, completely irrelevant. We had the immediate perception that something strange, but important, was happening. We put our food away, we took a video-camera, and after testing the neuron often enough to make sure that its response was not simply an artefact, we recorded the first mirror neuron. It was a *grasping-with-the-mouth-and-with-the-hand* mirror neuron. As in the case of the identities of both biter and sandwich, neither can the moniker 'mirror neuron' be attributed to one of us with enough certainty. I have the impression that maybe I was the inventor but, again, this is completely irrelevant. The last anecdotal report is related to Rizzolatti's first reaction to our finding. I remember he was not in Parma at the moment of the discovery, but on the day he came back, we all went into his room with the video of the mirror neuron. His first reaction was one of incredulity. But after watching the whole video, I clearly remember his sentence: 'If this is true, these neurons could provide a biological basis to Alvin Liberman's motor theory of speech perception!'.

The possible implications of mirror neurons are well described in the first part of this chapter. Our first paper on mirror neurons came out in experimental brain research (di Pellegrino et al., 1992, with our names in rigorously alphabetic order!) and the figures of this paper were drawn by Leonardo's wife, Giordana, who is a well-known artist (at least in our community!). Here I stress that, in my view, mirror neurons are *tools* for the brain, simply multipurpose tools that have nothing to do with fascinating issues like consciousness, theory of mind, or other very mentalistic concepts that have often been linked with them. Mirror neurons' discharge simply means that the representation of a given action is activated and this action representation is one of the contents of the observer's motor repertoire. In effect, the firing of mirror neurons represents the operation of an observation/ execution matching system for visually based actions. Mirror neurons do not provide our brain with the information that it is *another individual* that is moving and not ourselves; rather, other signals from different areas (e.g. proprioception, prefrontal activations) will perform this function. This apparent ambiguity (self v. other) of mirror neurons' discharge is shared by all visuo-motor (or even sensorimotor) neurons of the fronto-parietal circuits. Thus, a canonical neuron will discharge for the *presence* of a graspable object and during the *grasping action* of that same (or similar) object. A FEF (frontal eye field) visuo-motor neuron will respond equally during saccadic eye movement towards a given location and also to a visual stimulus that appears in that location, even in the absence of any ocular motion. A F4 bimodal sensorimotor neuron will respond when a physical stimulus is approaching our body surface and also when we move to reach out for it. This problem of the apparent ambiguity of sensorimotor responses is, to me, one of the most intriguing ones in neuroscience. I have devoted considerable time and thought to it, and I am convinced that sensorimotor responses are the best demonstration of the existence of motor representations, of potential motor acts and of motor ideas, which we evoke to interact with and interpret the world around us: objects, space and the actions of other people.

After our discovery of mirror neurons, I decided to follow two lines of research. The first was the investigation of the physiology of visuo-motor discharge in the monkey brain. To this purpose we devoted four years setting up a new monkey lab in Ferrara and conducting our first experiment, which is now ready for publication. The aim of the experiment was to test the hypothesis that mirror neurons might have evolved from another visual feedback system; specifically, the one that we use to control the precision and the accuracy of our actions. In this case, too, the brain has to solve the same problem it deals with in mirror neuron discharge, viewpoint independence, that is the independence of the visual response from the observer's physical point of view. Indeed, mirror neurons do not seem to be greatly influenced by the observer's perspective. This means that the implicit knowledge the brain has about a given action generalizes across the variability of the visual input into a 'point-of-view independent' visuo-motor representation. Now, thanks to our last monkey experiment, we know that the same happens during the visual control of one's own acting hand, and that a significant percentage of F5 motor neurons are indeed visuo-motor. They do not respond during the observation of another's actions, or during observation of graspable objects, but are sensitive to the *seeing* of one's own hand as it grasps something. I consider this a very promising field of research, maybe not so appealing for the media as the 'consciousness' and 'theory of mind' experiments done by several bright colleagues, but I am, and remain, a neurophysiologist.

My second line of research aims at demonstrating that humans have a mirror-neuron system too. This is not a trivial problem. Brain imaging experiments show that a specific network of parieto-frontal human areas are activated while looking at others' actions. However, they are so limited in temporal resolution that one cannot differentiate between brain activations resulting from observation of an action and subsequent activity associated with the actual performance of the observed motor act. How can we solve the problem of the specificity of the motor mirroring effect? More than 10 years ago I used transcranial magnetic stimulation (TMS) to investigate the motor excitability in the observer's brain. The advantage of TMS is that, when it is applied to the motor cortex, it makes an instantaneous map of the state of excitability of a brain region, detectable by electromyography such as motor-evoked potentials (MEPs). In brief, what we demonstrated in our *Journal of Neurophysiology* paper (Fadiga et al., 1995) is that if one observes another person closing their fingers onto an object (or even doing an intransitive movement), their hand MEPs (evoked by TMS on that hand's motor cortex) are specific and temporally congruent with the muscular state the observer would show if they were really doing the seen action. The finding that in humans intransitive movements are able to evoke a mirror effect, while in the monkey they do not, may provide a neurophysiological demonstration of our extremely developed capability to also imitate new, never before performed motor acts.

There is a final point that I would like to stress here. It concerns the link between action representation and language (in fact, I would rather say speech). This is not just a hypothetical association. It derives from the anatomical and cytoarchitectonic homologies linking the monkey area F5 (where we originally found the mirror neurons) and the human Broca's area, the motor centre for speech production (see Petrides et al., 2005). Again, by using TMS, we showed that the same effect found in the corticospinal system controlling the hand is also working for that controlling the tongue. When we listen to a speaker, our tongue's motor system becomes specifically facilitated and this can be revealed by TMS stimulation of the tongue motor cortex while recording motor-evoked potentials (MEPs) from tongue muscles. What it is different is the sensory part of the sensorimotor association (auditory v. visual) but, conceptually, the effect is equivalent. The finding that, during speech listening, our motor system mirrors the articulatory gestures used by the speaker to pronounce those words gives the first experimental support to Alvin Liberman's motor theory of speech perception. I met Professor Liberman twice. The last time I met him was at Riitta Hari's lab in Helsinki where, already quite old and close to the end of his days, he was still working like a student to carry out a magnetoencephaolgraphy (MEG) experiment on speech perception. Observing his enthusiasm, together with the statement by Giacomo Rizzolatti after the discovery of the mirror neurons, brings the story full circle in my view.

New challenges are now under way: one which I consider very interesting is our research on the link between the syntax of actions and the syntax of language. A further one is the hypothesis that Broca's area became a speech area because of its premotor origin. But this is another story. To be continued . . .

Peer commentary by Vilyanur S. Ramachandran

(Elements of the following appear in Ramachandran, V.S. Reflecting on the mind, *Nature*, 452: 814–15 (17 April 2008) | doi:10.1038/452814a, a book review of *Mirrors in the Brain* by Giacomo Rizzolatti and Corrado Sinigaglia. Translated by Frances Anderson. Oxford University Press: 2007.)

When a paradigm-shattering discovery is made in science, it goes through three stages before gaining acceptance. First, people do not believe it; second, they claim it is of no interest; and third, they say that they have always known it. The discovery of mirror neurons in the early 1990s by Giacomo Rizzolatti, Vittorio Gallese, Marco Iacoboni and others has been through all three stages. Happily, the idea seems to have emerged unscathed.

The paper under discussion here was one of their first to report the phenomenon of mirror neurons, a discovery that was made while studying the neural circuits in the brain that are involved in simple goal-directed movements. When a monkey reaches for a fruit or puts something in its mouth, motor-command neurons in area F5 in the frontal lobes fire. Different neurons fire for different actions. The team discovered that some of these motor-command neurons fire even when a monkey just watches another monkey performing the same action. He called these cells 'mirror neurons'. They allow one monkey to simulate or imagine another monkey's impending action. Mirror neurons have also been found that fire when a monkey watches another monkey being touched. Another class, canonical neurons, fire both when orchestrating the precise hand and finger movements required to grab a specific object and when one simply looks at that object. It is as if mere readiness to engage in a cylindrical grasp is synonymous – in terms of neural activity – with the perception of a cylinder.

Monitoring mirror-neuron activity might allow us to decipher the computations that lie at the elusive interface between perception and action, providing a key to understanding human cognition. If you extend the definition of action to include more abstract behavioural propensities, you could speak of the cells as representing 'meaning'. For example, an apple can conjure many ideas that neural activity may represent differently: it can be reached for and eaten, be used to tempt Eve, can keep the doctor away, go into a pie, and so on. Mirror neurons may also be involved in seemingly unrelated mental abilities, such as pretend play in children, imitating skilled actions, emotional empathy and constructing a useful model of another's actions to predict his or her intentions. Because these abilities are lost in autism, it has been suggested that the condition may result partly from mirror-neuron deficiency.

If a mirror neuron fires when someone touches you and when you watch someone being touched, how do you know the difference? One possibility is that when you watch someone else being touched, tactile receptors in your skin inform the regular, non-mirror neuron cells in your brain that they are not being touched, which inhibits the output of your mirror neurons. This would explain our observation that people who have had a hand amputated experience touch sensations in their phantom hand when watching another person's intact hand being touched. The absence of signals from the missing hand removes the inhibition, causing the patient to literally experience another person's sensations, dissolving the barrier between self and others. I have dubbed the cells involved here 'Gandhi neurons'. But the inhibition of mirror-neuron output by non-mirror neurons is not perfect even in people with no amputation, as first noted by Charles Darwin. He observed that we tend to unconsciously tense our calf muscles when watching someone getting ready to throw a javelin, for example.

We may have evolved mirror neurons or acquired them by associative learning. To explain the latter, every time the network that a neuron is part of sends a command, you see your hand moving; eventually, as a result of conditioning, the mere appearance of a moving hand (even someone else's) triggers the same neuron. This hypothesis cannot explain why regular, non-mirror, sensory neurons do not also develop such properties through associative conditioning. To explain this, one has to invoke a pre-existing, genetically specified scaffolding that imposes constraints on what is learned.

Infants imitate their mother smiling or sticking out her tongue, implying a mirror-neuron-like computation for translating the visual appearance into the sequence of muscle twitches. Learning cannot be involved because the infant has never seen its own face. It is possible that the infant's smile is just a reflex that does not require elaborate translation. This can be ruled out if the newborn can also mimic an asymmetrical smile or a peculiar expression, which demands a sophisticated interfacing between visual appearance and motor output.

Mirror neurons may also have clinical relevance for phantom pain and stroke rehabilitation. If a mirror is propped up vertically on a table in front of a patient with, for example, a paralysed left hand (so that one edge of the mirror is against his chest), the patient gets the illusion that the left hand is moving when he moves his right hand. We and others have found that this causes recovery from paralysis, perhaps by visually reviving dormant mirror neurons.

Some psychologists have criticized the idea of mirror neurons as being reductionist. Others think it is a mere metaphor for what psychologists have long called the 'theory of mind module' – the ability of our brains to construct internal models of other people's minds to predict their behaviour. This criticism reveals a fear that neuroscience might displace psychology ('neuron envy'), and a misunderstanding of reductionism. It is a bit like saying that the complementarity of the two strands of DNA is a metaphor for the complementarity of offspring and parent. Psychological and neural explanations are complementary, not mutually exclusive.

There has been a lot of media hype surrounding mirror neurons. The real danger is that too much is explained, not too little. This is inevitable with any new discovery but does not, in itself, vitiate the discovery's intrinsic importance. Nearly a decade ago, I wrote that 'mirror neurons will do for psychology what DNA did for biology'. It remains to be seen whether they will turn out to be anything as important as that, but as Sherlock Holmes said to Watson: 'The game is afoot'.

References

Broca, P. (1865) Sur le siége de la faculté du langage articulé, *Bulletin de la Société Anthropologique de Paris*, 6: 377–93.

di Pellegrino, G., Fadiga, L., Fogassi, L., Gallese, V. and Rizzolatti, G. (1992) Understanding motor events: a neurophysiological study, *Experimental Brain Research*, 91(1): 176–80.

Fadiga, L., Fogassi, L., Pavesi, G. and Rizzolatti, G. (1995) Motor facilitation during action observation: a magnetic stimulation study, *Journal of Neurophysiology*, 73(6): 2608–11.

Graziano, M.S., Hu, X.T. and Gross, C.G. (1997) Coding the locations of objects in the dark, *Science*, 277(5323): 190–1.

Petrides, M., Cadoret, G. and Mackey, S. (2005) Orofacial somatomotor responses in the macaque monkey homologue of Broca's area, *Nature*, 435(7046): 1235–8.

Rizzolatti, G., Camarda, R., Fogassi, L., Gentilucci, M., Luppino, G. and Matelli, M. (1988) Functional organization of inferior area 6 in the macaque monkey. II. Area F5 and the control of distal movements, *Experimental Brain Research*, 71(3): 491–507.

Rizzolatti, G. and Fadiga, L. (1998) Grasping objects and grasping action meanings: the dual role of monkey rostroventral premotor cortex (area F5), *Novartis Foundation Symposium*, 218: 81–95.

Rizzolatti, G., Fadiga, L., Fogassi, L. and Gallese, V. (1997) The space around us, *Science*, 277(5323): 239–41.

4   Cognition beyond perception: higher processing despite spatial neglect

Discussion of:

Vallar, G., Daini, R. and Antonucci, G. (2000)

Processing of illusion of length in spatial hemineglect: a study of line bisection, *Neuropsychologia*, 38(7): 1087–97

Reprinted with permission from Elsevier © 2000

Foreword, background and description by Richard A.P. Roche and Seán Commins
Author's commentary by Giuseppe Vallar
Peer commentary by Gereon Fink

Foreword

In this chapter, a paper is discussed that investigates aspects of the neuropsychological condition of unilateral spatial neglect, a severely disabling disorder, which typically follows damage to the right posterior–inferior parietal lobe, at the temporo-parietal junction. The study employs an ingenious design wherein a visual perceptual illusion, a variant of the classic Müller–Lyer illusion, is presented in part in the side of visual space that these patients neglect, typically the left-hand side in right-brain-damaged patients. By exploring whether the illusion is still effective even when presented to an area of space that the patients cannot perceive, we gain an insight into the fate of information that falls into the neglected region of the visual field.

Introduction

Our reality is more fragile than we often assume. While it may feel intuitively that the things that make up our world are objective, intransient and the same for everybody, evidence has repeatedly demonstrated the idiosyncratic nature of our reality and the factors that can influence our experience of it. The elements that constitute this experience, the things we perceive, feel, think and imagine, are based heavily on the structure of our brains, and the content of what we experience is critically dependent on the integrity of specific brain structures. In this chapter, we look at two areas in cognitive neuroscience that highlight the disparity that can exist between the objective contents of the environment and our own subjective experience of them. First, we consider the use of visual illusions in the study of human perception, and how the use of such illusions has advanced our understanding of the perceptual systems of the brain. Then we describe the neuropsychological syndrome of left spatial neglect following right parietal injury, and how this disorder impacts on its sufferers' experience of the visual environment. Finally, we turn to the paper under discussion in this chapter, that of Vallar et al. (2000), which combines these two elements to excellent effect in order to reveal aspects of processing in neglect patients.

In the early decades of cognitive psychology, one of the major debates that dominated the field concerned the extent to which human perception was driven by our knowledge and assumptions. Some argued that perception (and the majority of experimental investigations at the time focused on visual perception) was carried out in a 'top-down' manner, whereby the stimuli that entered the perceptual system from the environment were processed in the light of our stored knowledge of the world, our memories and expectations. In this way, the objective contents of the environment were thought to be filtered through the lens of our assumptions regarding how the world works to produce our subjective experience of reality. Principal evidence for this theoretical position came from the use of visual illusions of different types. Exponents of top-down processing argued that our automatic tendency to draw on stored knowledge when perceiving stimuli can lead us to make perceptual errors. For example, our experience of depth perception, they argued, leads us to perceive the top horizontal line as longer than the bottom one in the Ponzo Illusion (see Figure 4.1a), and the right vertical line as longer in the Müller–Lyer Illusion (Figure 4.1b). They claimed that this argued against those who championed the opposing, 'bottom-up' position, in which the two lines for comparison should be correctly perceived as the same length.

Further evidence for top-down processing came from our ability to accurately identify visual items (words, objects, etc.) in conditions when part of the item was obscured or occluded. Again, this tendency was shown to be subject to error, as in Figure 4.2, wherein our prior experience with a familiar phrase leads us to misread the actual contents of the visual environment (the presence of an extra 'the').

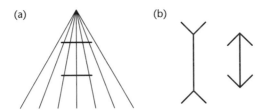

Figure 4.1 (a) The Ponzo Illusion, in which the top line is typically perceived as longer than the bottom line, and (b) the Müller–Lyer Illusion, in which the left line is perceived as longer than the right. Both effects are theorized to be due to our stored knowledge of depth perspective.

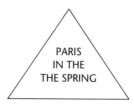

Figure 4.2 Familiarity with the phrase 'Paris in the spring' leads us to perceive this common phrase rather than the actual visual stimulus, which reads nonsensically 'Paris in the the spring'.

As is often the case in such theoretical debates, it was eventually conceded that both views held some merit: both top-down and bottom-up styles of processing appear to take place at different times and under different conditions. Significantly, however, the use of visual illusions such as the Ponzo and the Müller–Lyer revealed the subjective and error-prone nature of the human perceptual system, and provided an array of useful tools for those interested in how perceptual processing takes place.

A second area that emphasizes the fragility of human perception, and in particular its reliance on the integrity of the brain, is the study of left spatial neglect following right parietal cortical damage. The right parietal lobe is a common site of injury following stroke due to the unfortunate tendency of the right middle cerebral artery, the primary blood vessel in this region, towards infarct. Typical symptoms following right hemispheric stroke include motor and sensory impairments of the left side of the body (hemiplegia and hemianaesthesia), and left visual half-field deficits (hemianopia). However, in a number of patients, right parietal damage can result in the syndrome of left spatial or hemi-spatial neglect (also referred to as hemi-neglect). This syndrome, which may be found in about one-third to two-thirds of right-brain-damaged stroke patients, is characterized by an inability to report visual stimuli that are presented in the left side of the visual field. These patients also fail to explore the side of space contralateral to the cerebral lesion, and are therefore impaired in tasks requiring the crossing-out of targets, such as circles of letters, and in drawing tasks both by copy and from memory. Items presented in the neglected hemifield are ignored by the patient, as if they were not present, as can be seen in Figure 4.3, which shows attempts by a neglect patient to copy simple drawings. Figure 4.4 shows a series of self portraits by artist and neglect patient Anton Räderscheidt following a stroke, in which information to be laid down in the left-hand side of the painting is clearly omitted.[1] Since patients with left neglect are free to move their head and eyes in drawing and painting tasks, and patients with left hemianopia without neglect do not show this type of impairment, it is widely accepted that the dysfunction is an attentional one, rather than a visual deficit.

Neglect is a severely disabling disorder. Right-brain-damaged patients with left spatial neglect fail to perceive items on the left side of a dinner plate, leaving half the meal uneaten, as well as only shaving or dressing on the right side. They often misjudge the width of doorways and bump into the right side of the frame. Most interestingly,

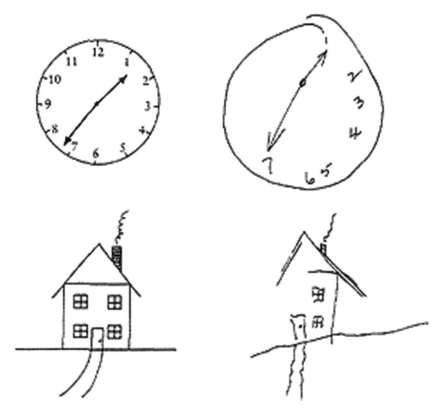

Figure 4.3 Attempts by a neglect patient to copy drawings of a clock and a house. Note how information from the left side of space is largely omitted.

Source: Image accessed from: www.plato.stanford.edu/entries/mental-imagery/
representational-neglect.html

the deficit even appears to extend to memories – a study by Bisiach and Luzzatti (1978) involved questioning Milanese neglect patients on the contents of the *Piazza Del Duomo* in Milan, Italy. When they were asked to recall the contents of the square while imagining standing with their back to a given side, they could only recall landmarks to their right. When asked to imagine standing at the opposite side, they were able to identify the features that they had previously neglected since they were no longer occupying the left neglected hemifield (of 'remembered space'). This last demonstration poses a fascinating question – what exactly happens to the information that is neglected? It would appear from the Piazza study that the complete contents of the square are all stored in the memory system, but only information on the right side of space (relative to the patient's imagined vantage position) can be accessed. If this is the case, then it argues strongly for the attentional interpretation of the deficit in hemineglect, suggesting that information from this hemifield is processed to a high level in the brain, and it is only a later stage of attentional selection that brings the information into conscious awareness.

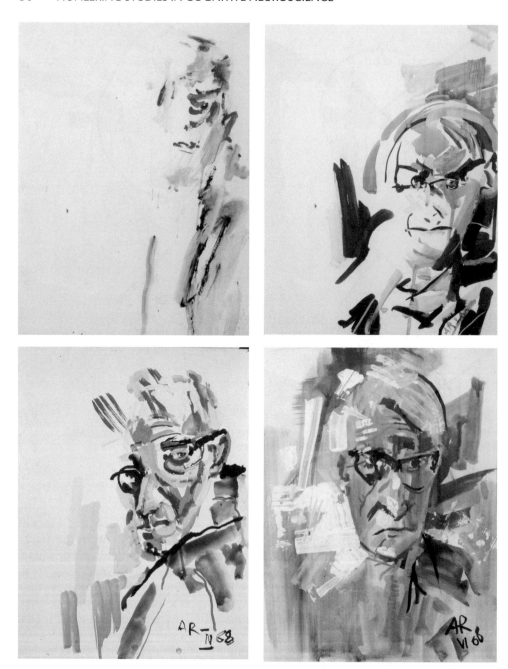

Figure 4.4 Self-portraits by German artist Anton Räderscheidt (1892–1970) following right parietal stroke. Information from the left side of space is largely omitted. These portraits were produced at different times following his stroke, and show some recovery of function over time as more information from the left visual field is included.

Source: Image accessed from: www-psych.stanford.edu/~lera/psych115s/notes/lecture15/figures.html

The Vallar et al. (2000) study that we discuss next combines these two areas to excellent effect by asking a group of neglect patients to complete a line bisection task incorporating a variant of the Müller–Lyer Illusion. The study capitalizes on a well-known impairment shown by neglect patients, who, when required to set the subjective midpoint of a horizontal line in a line bisection task, displace it to the *right* of the objective midpoint, as if they were underestimating the leftward extent of the line, in the neglected side of space. The Brentano form of the Müller–Lyer illusion utilizes inward- and outward-going arrowheads to manipulate the perceived length of parts of a horizontal line, thereby making one end of the line seem longer or shorter. If neglect patients' perceptions of line length can be manipulated in a similar manner to normal controls, *even when the illusion is presented in the neglected field*, then it will be compelling evidence for preserved processing to very high levels in neglect, despite a lack of conscious awareness of the information being processed.

Background and description of the study

Six patients suffering from left spatial neglect were used as participants. All were right-handed, had normal or corrected-to-normal vision and showed no evidence of psychiatric disorders or dementia. Six matched control participants were also used. These participants were also right-handed and had a mean age of 62.67 years with no history or evidence of neurological damage. Neuroimaging analyses of the right hemisphere lesions of the six patients revealed extensive damage to areas including the inferior parietal lobule, the superior temporal gyrus, the posterior region of the middle and inferior temporal gyri, pre-motor and opercular frontal cortices. Damage to these regions is known to bring about visuo-spatial neglect.

Initially, the authors conducted a series of neuropsychological baseline tests, in order to assess that the patients were indeed suffering from left spatial neglect. Tests included visuo-exploratory tasks (the line cancellation test; Albert, 1978), the letter cancellation test (Diller and Weinberg, 1977), a sentence reading test, and the Wundt–Jastrow illusion test (Massironi, 1988). For example, in the line cancellation test, participants are given a sheet of paper with lines of various orientations (Figure 4.5a). Patients are asked to cross out every line on the page. Those with right hemisphere damage should make more omissions on the left-hand side of the sheet, in the side contralateral to the hemispheric lesion (Figure 4.5b).

Results from these tests confirmed that all six patients suffered from left spatial neglect. In the line cancellation test, for example, the scores for the number of crossed targets on the right-hand side of the sheet (intact hemifield) were 10/10, 9/10, 9/10, 8/10, 9/10 and 10/10 for each of the six patients. This compares to their performance on the *left-hand side* of the sheet (neglected hemifield), which was 7/11, 0/11, 0/11, 0/11, 3/11 and 3/11. Results from the other tests followed a similar pattern.

Following these neuropsychological tests, Vallar et al., in their first experiment, presented both the patient group and the control group with stimuli that consisted of a Brentano version of the Müller–Lyer illusion (see Figure 4.6; Coren and Girgus, 1978). These stimuli were presented on an A4 sheet of paper placed directly in front of

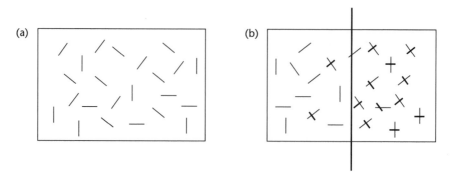

Figure 4.5 (a) Line cancellation task stimuli as presented to participants, and (b) following task completion by a hemi-neglect patient.

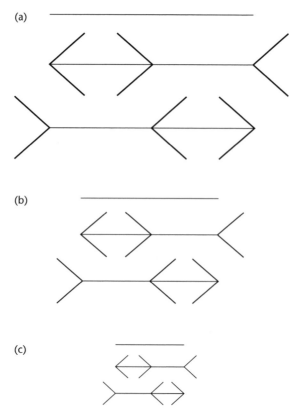

Figure 4.6 Stimuli. Simple line, and the Brentano form of the Müller–Lyer illusion with right-sided and left-sided outgoing fins (a), (b), and (c) show stimuli 24, 16 and 8 cm in length.

Source: Reprinted by permission from Elsevier: *Neuropsychologia* (Vallar et al., 2000), © (2000).

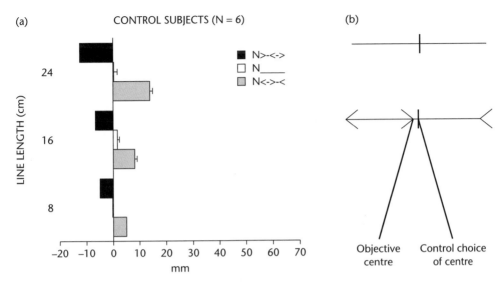

Figure 4.7 (a) Mean transaction displacements and standard errors of control subjects by line length (8, 16 and 24 cm) and stimulus type (simple line, right-sided outgoing fin, left-sided outgoing fin); (b) representative response by control participants.

Source: Reprinted by permission from Elsevier: *Neuropsychologia* (Vallar et al., 2000), © (2000).

each participant (with the centre of the stimulus being aligned to the mid-sagittal plane of the trunk of the body). The first stimulus consisted of a simple straight line (top line in Figure 4.6a, b and c), the second with right-side outgoing fin/left-sided ingoing fin (middle line in Figure 4.6a, b and c) and the third with left-sided outgoing fin/right-sided ingoing fin (bottom line in Figure 4.6a, b and c). The stimuli lengths varied in size between 24 cm, 16 cm and 8 cm (Figure 4.6a, b and c, respectively). In the first experiment, each participant simply had to mark with a pen where they perceived the middle of the horizontal line was located. They were not given any instructions about the fins. Deviations in millimetres from the objective midpoint of the horizontal line was used to score the patients' performance (a negative score indicated a deviation to the left, a positive score deviation to the right).

Results indicated that the control group had little difficulty in marking the midpoint of the simple straight line, with the length of the line also having no effect (Figure 4.7a (white bars) and 4.7b upper line). In the case of the right-sided outgoing fin (middle line in Figure 4.6a, b and c), control participants tended to place the mark slightly to the right of the objective centre and this right bias seemed to increase with increasing size of the line (Figure 4.7a (grey bars) and 4.7b lower line). In the case of the left-sided outgoing fin (bottom line in Figure 4.6a, b and c), the opposite was the case, with a leftward bias that also increased with the length of the line (Figure 4.7a black bars).

Results from the neglect group showed that, in the simple line condition, the greater the line length the greater the displacement to the right (Figure 4.8, white bars).

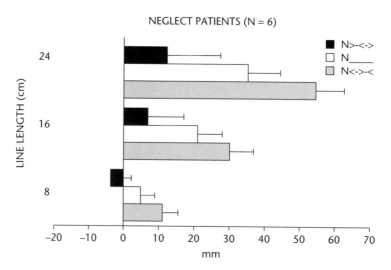

Figure 4.8 (a) Mean transaction displacements and standard errors of hemi-neglect patients by line length (8, 16 and 24 cm) and stimulus type (simple line, right-sided outgoing fin, left-sided outgoing fin).

Source: Reprinted with permission from Elsevier: *Neuropsychologia* (Vallar et al., 2000), © (2000).

This was in contrast to the control group above that did not show an effect of line length. In the case of the right-sided outgoing fin (Figure 4.8, grey bars), neglect patients placed the mark significantly more to right of the objective centre compared to the control group. In addition, and similar to the control participants, this right bias increased with line length. For the left-sided outgoing fin condition, there was a small but significant effect of line length (Figure 4.8, black bars) with a slight rightward bias. Therefore in both of the illusionary conditions (right- and left-sided outgoing fins), the control group and the patient group performed similarly. Both groups were affected by line length and both showed the illusion directionality effect (although the neglect patients demonstrated a general rightward shift, as would be expected). However, in the simple line condition, there was a dissociation between the two groups. The patient group showed an increasing rightward bias with increasing line length. This was not observed in the control group.

Using a new set of control participants ($n = 6$), but keeping the same patient group, Vallar and colleagues then conducted a second experiment to see if there was an effect of the position and location of the stimulus. The same stimuli used in Experiment 1 were employed for this experiment. However, rather then placing the stimulus directly in front of each participant (as in Experiment 1), the stimuli were positioned either to the left, centred or to the right of the mid-sagittal plane of the trunk of each participant. That is, in the left condition, the right end on the line was aligned with the centre of each participant's body trunk (Figure 4.9a), in the right condition, the left end on the line was aligned with the centre of the participant's body trunk (Figure 4.9b), and in the centre condition the stimulus was directly aligned with the

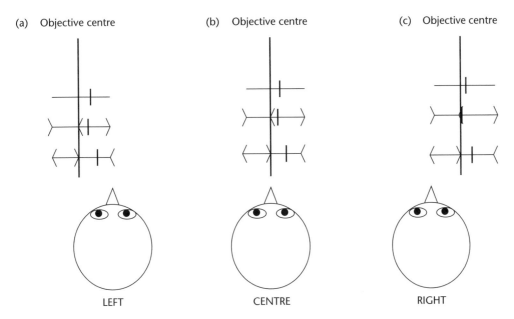

(a)   Objective centre   (b)   Objective centre   (c)   Objective centre

LEFT   CENTRE   RIGHT

Figure 4.9 Representative responses sorted by stimulus type and spatial position of the stimulus (a, b and c) for hemi-neglect patients.

Source: Reprinted with permission from Elsevier: *Neuropsychologia* (Vallar et al., 2000), © (2000).

participant's body trunk (Figure 4.9c). Again three different line lengths were used (8 cm, 16 cm and 24 cm).

Results indicated that the control participants showed similar illusory effects to those reported in Experiment 1, with a rightward bias that increased with line length for the illusion with the right outgoing fin (Figure 4.10, grey bars) and a leftward bias that also increased with line length for the illusion with the left outgoing fin (Figure 4.10, black bars). Again similar to Experiment 1, there was no effect for the simple line (Figure 4.10, white bars). In addition to these results, there was no effect of stimulus positioning for any condition or any line length (Figure 4.10, comparisons of right, centre and left conditions).

The patient group also showed similar effects to the illusions as reported in the first experiment, with a rightward bias that was stronger than in the control group, for the right outgoing fin (Figure 4.11, grey bars). This bias increased with line length for the illusion. Similarly, patients showed a small effect for the illusion with the left outgoing fin with a slight bias to the right as the line increased in length (Figure 4.11, black bars). Again similar to Experiment 1 (and in contrast to the control group) there was a length effect for the simple line (Figure 4.11, white bars) with a significant rightward bias. Interestingly (and again in contrast to the control group), there was a significant effect for the position of the stimulus. In the right position, the rightward bias was small, but as the stimulus moved towards the centre and the left position, there were significant increases in the rightward bias.

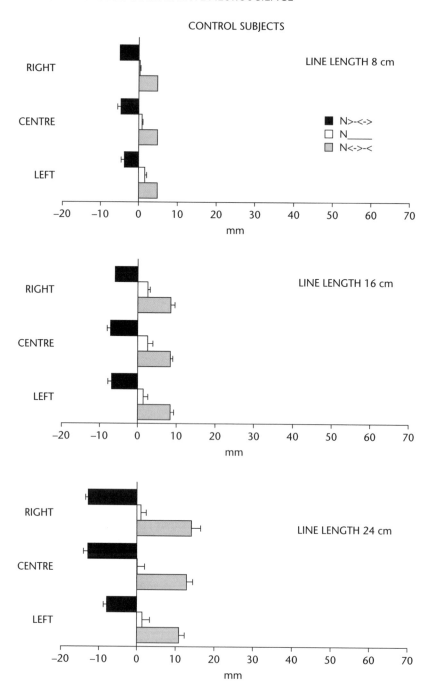

Figure 4.10 Mean transaction errors and standard errors, by line length and stimulus type, and spatial position of the stimulus (right, centre, left) for control participants.

Source: Reprinted with permission from Elsevier: *Neuropsychologia* (Vallar et al., 2000), © (2000).

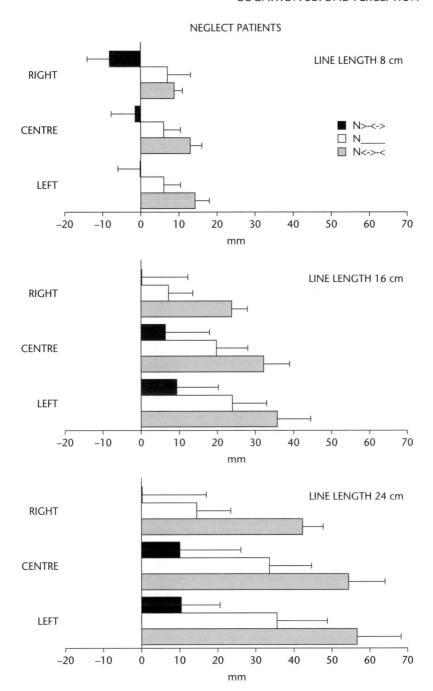

Figure 4.11 Mean transaction errors and standard errors, by line length and stimulus type, and spatial position of the stimulus (right, centre, left) for hemi-neglect patients.

Source: Reprinted with permission from Elsevier: *Neuropsychologia* (Vallar et al., 2000), © (2000).

Author commentary by Giuseppe Vallar

When this study (Vallar et al., 2000), henceforth the '2000' study, was performed, I was Professor of Psychology at the University of Roma 'La Sapienza', researching brain-damaged patients in the 'IRCCS Fondazione S. Lucia' in Roma, a well-known centre dedicated to the rehabilitation of brain-damaged patients, and to both basic and applied clinical research in the field. My main interest, both at that time and indeed at present, was the fascinating syndrome of unilateral spatial neglect. I had been introduced to its mysteries and multifarious intriguing manifestations by my former professor and 'maestro', Edoardo Bisiach (Marshall and Vallar, 2004), who, in the 1970s and early 1980s, was Associate Professor of Neurology at the University of Milano, Italy, and an eminent figure in the Centro di Neuropsicologia of the Neurological Department (Grossi and Boller, 1996). Having completed my MD degree (1976), later specializing in neurology (1980), I went on to work as a Research Assistant in the Neurological Department. My research concerned phonological short-term (working) memory (Vallar and Baddeley, 1984), and the neuroanatomy of unilateral spatial neglect (Vallar and Perani, 1986).

The contributions of Edoardo Bisiach, who retired a few years ago, to our understanding of the neglect syndrome are manifold. Perhaps his most pertinent contribution to the '2000' study (Bisiach and Vallar, 2000) was his convincing demonstration that spatial neglect is a disorder of the conscious internal representation of space, and that this representation is *corrupted* or *truncated* in the left side, contralateral to the damaged right hemisphere, leaving it unavailable to conscious phenomenal experience (Berti, 2004). This representational approach, with the core deficit of neglect being the defective access to conscious experience of left-sided information, makes allowance for the possibility that neglected information *may be* processed by the nervous system implicitly, up to and including the extraction of its meaning. And many studies in brain-damaged patients (using a variety of tasks including semantic priming, optional choice and reading) have indeed shown that this is the case (see Berti, 2002, for a review).

In 1992 I moved to Rome, to become Associate, and then full Professor of Psychology at the University of Roma 'La Sapienza', joining a very active group of neuropsychologists led by Professor Luigi Pizzamiglio in the 'IRCCS Fondazione S. Lucia'. Pizzamiglio's team was increasingly interested in unilateral spatial neglect, particularly in the then novel field of its rehabilitation (Pizzamiglio et al., 1992, 2006). Another main topic of Pizzamiglio's group was visual perception. So, in collaboration with two psychologists (Gabriella Antonucci and Roberta Daini) who were interested in visual perception, I started discussing the possibility of investigating the processing of visual illusions of length by patients with left hemineglect (see Zoccolotti et al., 1997). The basic idea was to assess whether left spatial unilateral neglect disrupted the processing of illusions of length. There was some evidence from studies using the Müller–Lyer (Mattingley et al., 1995, with seven patients), and the Judd (Ro and Rafal, 1996, with one patient) illusions that right-brain-damaged patients suffering from left neglect may show illusory effects in tasks requiring the bisection of horizontal segments, both leftwards, towards the neglected side of space, and rightwards. The observation of preserved illusory effects (*illusions in neglect*), even when the illusion arises in the left-hand side of the display, suggests that such phenomena are *pre-attentive*; therefore, the spatial neglect which affects the contralesional orientation of spatial attention does not prevent or preclude the processing of illusions in this hemifield.

We used the Brentano version of the Müller–Lyer illusion (Coren and Gircus, 1978), which was suitable for investigating the lateral asymmetry of unilateral spatial neglect, combining (as does the Judd illusion) an illusory expansion on one side (either the left or the right) with a compression on the other. Results showed the complete preservation of the illusory effects both on the right-hand side of the figure, and, importantly, on the left-hand side, even when the whole of the stimulus was placed in the left-hand (i.e. neglected) side of space with respect to the mid-sagittal plane of the subject's trunk. Under these conditions, the rightward bisection error that characterizes left neglect worsened, as expected (Heilman and Valenstein, 1979), but the illusory effects did not change. The independence of spatial neglect on the one hand, and of the illusory effects on the other, is well illustrated by some anecdotal observations made by one of us (Roberta Daini). Often, right-brain-damaged patients with left neglect verbally reported the presence of the right-sided, and central fins, but not those on the left side before performing the bisection task. Furthermore, patients sometimes explored the right-hand side of the Brentano–Müller–Lyer figure with their right index finger but not the left-hand side. Notwithstanding these verbal reports and patterns of visuo-motor exploration that may indicate the presence of left neglect for the fins themselves, the patients' bisection performance showed preserved effects of the *illusion* in the neglected side.

Similar findings had been reported more systematically by Ro and Rafal (Judd illusion: 1996) in one right-brain-damaged patient, and these effects were later confirmed in a group study by Olk and coworkers (Müller–Lyer and Judd illusions: Olk et al., 2001). The dissociation between these fully preserved illusory effects on the one hand, and the patients' inability to perform explicit perceptual judgements involving the left-sided fins (and sometimes even to report them) on the other hand, supports the view that the Brentano–Müller–Lyer effects do not involve the processes of conscious awareness supported by spatial attention and representation that are defective in patients with left neglect.

Illusions of length such as the Müller–Lyer figure and its variants are also of interest in another important respect. In neurologically unimpaired participants, illusory configurations that expand the perceived extent of the horizontal shaft rightwards (with a relative 'compression' of its left-sided extent) bring about a rightward directional error (i.e. the right side of the line is perceived as longer and so participants will bisect the line further to the right). This mimics the error committed by right-brain-damaged patients with left neglect. Conversely, configurations that expand the perceived extent of the horizontal shaft *leftwards* (with a relative 'compression' of its right-sided extent) bring about a leftward error, mirroring the rightward error committed by right-brain-damaged patients with left neglect (see also Fleming and Behrmann, 1998).

These *illusions of neglect* (Vallar and Daini, 2002) provide some insight into the pathological mechanisms of the syndrome. Particularly, they support the view that the ipsilesional, rightward error committed by these patients in line bisection may reflect a perceptual underestimation of the contralesional, leftward part of the segment that is 'seen' with the 'mind's eyes' as shorter. This interpretation may also account for the observation, made by Milner and Harvey (1995), that patients with left neglect underestimate the lateral extent of left-sided 2D configurations such as rectangles, compared with right-sided configurations. This finding has been confirmed by a number of successive studies (e.g. Irving-Bell et al., 1999; Kerkhoff, 2000), and also in the tactile modality (Pritchard et al., 2001). The underestimation of lateral extent, however, may also be brought about by a rare perceptual (non-spatial) disorder termed 'hemimicropsia' (see Frassinetti et al.,

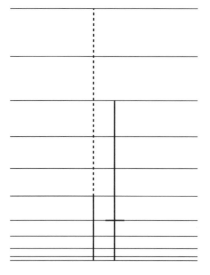

Figure 4.12 Horizontal anisometry of the medium for the representation of spatial relationships (modified from Bisiach and Vallar, 2000). Contralesional relaxation of the medium for space representation causing rightward bisection error (above) and left overextension (below, dotted line).

Bisiach, E., Vallar, G.: Unilateral neglect in humans. In Boller, F. and Grafman, J. (eds). Handbook of neuropsychology. Amsterdam: Elsevier, pp. 459–502, 2000.

1999 for a patient with horizontal dysmetropsia), in which patients see objects disproportionately smaller in size (see also Ferber and Karnath, 2001).

Figure 4.12 shows a schematic representation of the illusion of Oppel–Kundt (Watt, 1994) that brings about an expansion/compression of the perceived lateral extent of a segment. As Figure 4.12 shows, a denser background illusorily expands the perceived length of the horizontal segment. Conversely, a wider background shortens the perceived length of the horizontal segment. In order to simulate left spatial neglect, the wider background in Figure 4.12 is on the left-hand side, and the denser one on the right-hand side. As with the Brentano version of the Müller–Lyer figure, experiments in brain-damaged patients using the Oppel–Kundt illusion have also been performed. The line bisection performance of right-brain-damaged patients with left neglect is also influenced by the Oppel–Kundt illusion, with both a left- and a right-sided denser background (Ricci et al., 2004), corroborating the finding that illusions of lateral extent in the neglected side of space may both be processed, and may affect motor performance in the bisection task.

The model shown in Figure 4.12 may also account for the observation that, when required to set the two ends of a line given its mid-point (Bisiach et al., 1994; Bisiach et al., 1996), or to reproduce the length of a segment doubling its original length (line extension task: Bisiach et al., 1998), right-brain-damaged patients produce, paradoxically, longer extents when a leftward movement is required (i.e. towards the neglected left side). Later studies have shown that visual field deficits (haemianopia) may play a relevant role in bringing about the disproportionate contralesional extension made by right-brain-damaged patients with left neglect (Doricchi and Angelelli, 1999; Doricchi et al., 2003). Furthermore, a disproportionate contralesional extension, as found in the spontaneous drawing of putatively symmetrical objects such as a daisy, has been reported in right-brain-damaged patients with no evidence of left haemianopia and spatial neglect (Rode et al., 2006; Rode et al., 2008). In sum, the contralesional disproportionate expansion of the spatial medium, simulated by the Oppel–Kundt illusion, has proved to be a real pathological impairment of some right-brain-damaged patients. The deficit, however, may be independent of left spatial neglect.

The '2000' study stimulated further experiments aimed at defining more precisely the neural underpinnings of the Brentano version of the Müller–Lyer illusion. In a later study

(Daini et al., 2002), we found that right-brain-damaged patients with both left neglect and left visual half-field deficits were insensitive to the illusory effects on the left side. These patients' lesions were more posterior (involving the occipital lobes), however, than those of right-brain-damaged patients who exhibited the illusory effects. Similar results have been recently reported for the Oppel–Kundt illusion (Savazzi et al., 2007; see also Vuilleumier and Landis, 1998, 2001). These neuropsychological findings have been confirmed and extended by a recent fMRI experiment in neurologically unimpaired participants (Weidner and Fink, 2007). A task requiring participants to judge whether the central fin correctly bisects the horizontal line of the Brentano–Müller–Lyer figure was compared to a landmark task requiring a similar judgment on a pre-bisected simple line.

For the illusory stimulus, which is of interest here, activations were found bilaterally in the lateral occipital extrastriate cortex, particularly in the inferior occipital gyrus, and also in the superior end of the right superior parietal lobule (SPL). The activation in the lateral occipital cortex (a region whose damage is not typically associated with unilateral spatial neglect) is compatible with the neuropsychological data from the '2000' study. Consistent with these findings, there is evidence from a study using repetitive transcranial magnetic stimulation (TMS) that the extrastriate visual cortex is involved in the processing of illusory contours (Brighina et al., 2003). It should be noted, however, that a unilateral lesion involving the occipital lobes or the optic radiations (bringing about a contralateral hemianopia *without neglect*) does not abolish the Brentano–Müller–Lyer illusory effects, either contralesionally or ipsilesionally. The illusion is likely to be processed appropriately, because these brain-damaged patients (with hemianopia but without neglect) are able to explore both sides of the figure, therefore compensating for the hemianopia by means of their contralateral, undamaged, occipital lobe (Daini et al., 2002).

Finally, the activation of the right SPL found by Weidner and Fink (2007) may be interpreted in terms of an interaction between the parietal and the lateral occipital regions (possibly with parietal top-down processes). In line with these findings, we (Daini et al., 2002) found that the illusory effects towards the left/neglected side were not only preserved, but even disproportionately increased. We suggest that the fronto-temporo-parietal lesions typically bringing about unilateral spatial neglect (Halligan et al., 2003) may also disrupt ipsilesional, top-down modulation processes (possibly attentional-based), which are exerted on the occipital regions responsible for the illusory effects. These modulation effects may be inhibitory in nature, with their disruption bringing about larger illusory effects. The finding that the magnitude of the Brentano–Müller–Lyer illusion decreases with age (Predebon, 1984) may be also interpreted in this light, possibly attributable to the modulation of attentional or executive systems.

In conclusion, the '2000' study first reveals a domain of visuo-spatial processing that is spared in right-brain-damaged patients with left neglect. This concerns a preserved representation of lateral extent, as indexed by the effects of the Brentano–Müller–Lyer illusion. The task used in the '2000' study, namely line bisection, appears to probe processes that do not involve conscious spatial attentional and representational systems, since patients may be unable to report the left-sided fins, or make perceptual judgements on them, but still exhibit preserved illusory effects. Second, the Brentano–Müller–Lyer illusion provides a simulation of some aspects of spatial neglect, elucidating some putative pathological mechanisms. Third, the '2000' study provides some evidence about the neural underpinnings of the Brentano–Müller–Lyer illusion, which have been subsequently confirmed and further defined by imaging experiments in neurologically unimpaired participants.

Peer commentary by Gereon R. Fink

Neglect is a disorder of spatial attention that generally follows fronto-temporo-parietal damage and results in the patient's failure to report or even orient to stimuli occurring on the side of space contralateral to the lesion (Halligan et al., 2003). Similarly, the syndrome of extinction, often viewed as a mild form of neglect and often seen following recovery from severe forms of spatial neglect, results from a difficulty in reporting contralesional stimuli when an ipsilateral stimulus is presented simultaneously. The behaviour of patients suffering from either neglect or extinction suggests that they do not perceive the neglected or extinguished stimuli. However, evidence has been accumulated over the last two decades that shows that, at least in some patients suffering from neglect or extinction, the neglected or extinguished stimuli get processed right to the level of meaning despite the lack of (explicit) awareness.

In a variety of neurological syndromes, patients may show tacit awareness of stimuli that cannot be consciously recollected or identified. For example, such dissociations are the defining characteristic of 'blindsight' (see Chapter 6); however, comparable dissociations between overt and covert perception have also been reported in patients suffering from visuo-spatial neglect (Marshall and Halligan, 1988). In another seminal paper, Marshall and Halligan reported that their patient P.S. had sustained right cerebral damage and failed overtly to process information in the contralesional hemispace. In common with many patients who manifest left-sided neglect, P.S. also suffered from left homonymous hemianopia. Nonetheless, P.S.'s neglect persisted despite free movements of the head and eyes and was thus not a direct consequence of sensory loss in the left visual field. Marshall and Halligan presented P.S. simultaneously with two line drawings of a house, in one of which the left side was on fire. P.S. judged that the drawings were identical; yet when asked to select which house she would prefer to live in, she reliably chose the house that was not burning.

The study by Vallar et al. considerably adds to the notion that in a neglect patient information can be processed to the level of meaning despite the lack of awareness for the stimuli. In their seminal paper, Vallar et al. used a visual perceptual illusion presented in part in the the neglected (hemi-)space to provide clear-cut evidence that information that is neglected can nevertheless be processed to the level of meaning and hence impact on the patient's behaviour (Vallar et al., 2000). An illusion is a distortion of the senses, revealing how the brain normally organizes and interprets sensory stimulation. Importantly, while illusions distort reality, they are *generally* shared by most people. Illusions may occur with all human senses, but visual illusions are the most well known and understood. Some visual illusions are based on general assumptions our brains make during perception. These assumptions are made based on general organizational principles, like *Gestalt*, an individual's ability of depth perception and motion perception, or perceptual constancy.

An optical illusion is characterized by visually perceived images that, at least in common-sense terms, convey deceptive or misleading information. Therefore, the visual information gathered is processed by the brain to give, on the face of it, a percept that does not tally with a physical measurement of the stimulus. A common notion is that there are physiological illusions that occur naturally and cognitive illusions that can be demonstrated by specific visual tricks that say something more basic about how human perceptual systems work. In other words, the human brain constructs a world inside our head based on what it samples from the surrounding environment *interpreted* on the basis of prior knowledge. It then tries to organize this information as it thinks best while at other times it fills in gaps/missing information ('perceptual filling'). These processes are at the core of an illusion.

The really clever idea of Vallar and colleagues was that they made use of a well-known illusion to learn more about the perceptual processing both in normal subjects and the fate of such information in patients suffering from visuo-spatial neglect. Arrows terminating a line can distort the perceived line length. This so-called Müller–Lyer illusion can be used in healthy subjects to mimic the performance of neglect patients in visuo-spatial judgements (e.g. in the landmark task, i.e. the Brentano version of the Müller–Lyer illusion): healthy subjects misperceive the length of one segment of a pre-bisected line and hence misjudge the line bisection. Vallar and colleagues investigated both normal subjects and neglect patients and were able to show that, despite the similarity between the illusion-induced impairment of a visuo-spatial judgement and the performance of neglect patients, the two phenomena seem to have different origins: The illusory effects induced by the Müller–Lyer figures can be preserved in patients with visuo-spatial neglect (Ro and Rafal, 1996) and these effects persist irrespective of the illusion-inducing arrows being presented within or outside the neglected visual hemifield (Vallar et al., 2000). Accordingly, Vallar and colleagues suggested that the neural structures involved in generating the Müller–Lyer illusion may reside in areas different from those which, when lesioned, may cause neglect, for example extrastriate cortex.

This suggestion inspired us to perform an imaging experiment since the hypothesis put forward by Vallar and his colleagues can be tested directly: using fMRI we investigated the neural mechanisms underlying the Müller–Lyer illusion, the landmark task, and their interaction (Weidner and Fink, 2007). This was achieved by parametrically manipulating the magnitude of the Müller–Lyer illusion both in a landmark and a luminance (control) task. As expected (e.g. Fink et al., 2000), the landmark task activated right posterior parietal cortex and right temporo-occipital cortex. In contrast, the neural processes associated with the strength of the Müller–Lyer illusion were located bilaterally in lateral occipital cortex as well as right superior parietal cortex. The data converge with but also extend neuropsychological data that indicate maintained line-length illusion in neglect patients. In addition, the results support the size-constancy scaling hypothesis (Gregory, 1968) as a putative mechanism underlying line-length illusions. Furthermore, activation that was driven by both the task as well as the strength of the Müller–Lyer illusion was observed in right intraparietal sulcus (IPS) thus arguing in favour of an interaction of illusory information with the top-down processes underlying visuo-spatial judgements in right parietal cortex. The data fit nicely with both neuropsychological work and other functional imaging studies that investigated the neural mechanisms underlying the processing of illusory information.

The seminal work by Vallar and colleagues is a fine example of a series of important studies performed by neuropsychologists who fruitfully combined basic psychological processes with the investigation of neuropsychological deficits. Other outstanding examples are the above-mentioned study by Marshall and Halligan (1998) on 'blindsight' in neglect or the investigation of Driver et al. (1992) of preserved figure-ground segmentation and symmetry perception in neglect. These studies laid the groundwork for many subsequent behavioural and functional imaging studies. They inspired fellow scientists and highlight the importance of combining studies of both normal subjects and patients thus exemplifying the bidirectional value of cognitive neuropsychology – informing both psychology/basic neuroscience and clinical neurology. The convergence of cognitive neuropsychological data with functional imaging data further strengthens the contributions made as it allows for testing directly the hypotheses generated from psychological and neuropsychological observations.

Note

1 Note also that the ability to perceive the left hemifield appears to return over time, as evidenced by the increased number of features in the left field as the time since stroke increases.

References

Albert, M.L. (1978) A simple test of visual neglect, *Neurology*, 23: 658–64.

Berti, A. (2002) Unconscious processing in neglect, in H.-O. Karnath, A.D. Milner and G. Vallar (eds) *The Cognitive and Neural Bases of Spatial Neglect*, pp. 313–26. Oxford: Oxford University Press.

Berti, A. (2004) Cognition in dyschiria: Edoardo Bisiach's theory of spatial disorders and consciousness, *Cortex*, 40: 275–80.

Bisiach, E., Pizzamiglio, L., Nico, D. and Antonucci, G. (1996) Beyond unilateral neglect, *Brain*, 119: 851–7.

Bisiach, E. and Luzzatti, C. (1978) Unilateral neglect of representational space, *Cortex*, 14(1): 129–33.

Bisiach, E. and Vallar, G. (2000) Unilateral neglect in humans, in F. Boller, J. Grafman and G. Rizzolatti (eds) *Handbook of Neuropsychology*, Vol. 1 (2nd edn.), pp. 459–502. Amsterdam: Elsevier Science, B.V.

Bisiach, E., Ricci, R. and Neppi Mòdona, M. (1998) Visual awareness and anisometry of space representation in unilateral neglect: a panoramic investigation by means of a line extension task, *Consciousness and Cognition*, 7: 327–55.

Bisiach, E., Rusconi, M.L., Peretti, V. and Vallar, G. (1994) Challenging current accounts of unilateral neglect, *Neuropsychologia*, 32: 1431–4.

Brighina, F., Ricci, R., Piazza, A. et al. (2003) Illusory contours and specific regions of human extrastriate cortex: evidence from rTMS, *European Journal of Neuroscience*, 17: 2469–74.

Coren, S. and Gircus, J.S. (1978) Visual illusions, in R. Held, H.W. Leibowitz and H.-L. Teuber (eds) *Handbook of Sensory Physiology: Perception*, Vol. 8, pp. 548–68. Heidelberg: Springer-Verlag.

Daini, R., Angelelli, P., Antonucci, G., Cappa, S.F. and Vallar, G. (2002) Exploring the syndrome of spatial unilateral neglect through an illusion of length, *Experimental Brain Research*, 144: 224–37.

Diller, L. and Weinberg, J. (1977) Hemi-inattention in rehabilitation: the evolution of a rational remediation program, in E.A. Weinstein and R.P. Friedland (eds) *Hemi-inattention and Hemisphere Specialization*, pp. 62–82. New York: Raven Press.

Doricchi, F. and Angelelli, P. (1999) Misrepresentation of horizontal space in left unilateral neglect: role of hemianopia, *Neurology*, 52: 1845–52.

Doricchi, F., Guariglia, P., Figliozzi, F., Magnotti, L. and Gabriele, G. (2003) Retinotopic modulation of space misrepresentation in unilateral neglect: evidence from quadrantanopia, *Journal of Neurology, Neurosurgery and Psychiatry*, 74: 116–19.

Driver, J., Baylis, G.C. and Rafal, R.D. (1992) Preserved figure-ground segregation and symmetry perception in visual neglect, *Nature*, 360: 73–5.

Ferber, S. and Karnath, H.-O. (2001) Size perception in hemianopia and neglect, *Brain*, 124: 527–36.

Fink, G.R., Marshall, J.C., Shah, N.J. et al. (2000) Line bisection judgements implicate right parietal cortex and cerebellum as assessed by fMRI, *Neurology*, 54: 1324–31.

Fleming, J. and Behrmann, M. (1998) Visuospatial neglect in normal subjects: altered spatial representations induced by a perceptual illusion, *Neuropsychologia*, 36: 469–75.

Frassinetti, F., Nichelli, P. and di Pellegrino, G. (1999) Selective horizontal dysmetropsia following prestriate lesion, *Brain*, 122: 339–50.

Gregory, R.L. (1968) Perceptual illusions and brain models, *Proceedings of the Royal Society of London Series B Biological Sciences*, 171: 279–96.

Grossi, D. and Boller, F. (1996) Sviluppo della neuropsicologia italiana moderna, in G. Denes and L. Pizzamiglio (eds) *Manuale di Neuropsicologia* (2nd edn.), pp. 16–34. Bologna: Zanichelli.

Halligan, P.W., Fink, G.R., Marshall, J.C. and Vallar, G. (2003) Spatial cognition: evidence from visual neglect, *Trends in Cognitive Sciences*, 7: 125–33.

Heilman, K.M. and Valenstein, E. (1979) Mechanisms underlying hemispatial neglect, *Annals of Neurology*, 5: 166–70.

Irving-Bell, L., Small, M. and Cowey, A. (1999) A distortion of perceived space in patients with right-hemisphere lesions and visual hemineglect, *Neuropsychologia*, 37: 919–25.

Kerkhoff, G. (2000) Multiple perceptual distortions and their modulation in leftsided visual neglect, *Neuropsychologia*, 38: 1073–86.

Marshall, J.C. and Halligan, P.W. (1988) Blindsight and insight in visuo-spatial neglect, *Nature*, 336: 766–7.

Marshall, J.C. and Vallar, G. (eds) (2004) *Spatial Neglect: A Representational Disorder? A Festschrift for Edoardo Bisiach*. The Cortex book series. Milan: Masson.

Massironi, M.A. (1988) A new visual problem: phenomenic folding, *Perception*, 17: 681–94.

Mattingley, J.B., Bradshaw, J.L. and Bradshaw, J.A. (1995) The effects of unilateral visuospatial neglect on perception of Müller–Lyer illusory figures, *Perception*, 24: 415–33.

Milner, A.D. and Harvey, M. (1995) Distortion of size perception in visuospatial neglect, *Current Biology*, 5: 85–9.

Olk, B., Harvey, M., Dow, L. and Murphy, P.J.S. (2001) Illusion processing in hemispatial neglect, *Neuropsychologia*, 39: 611–25.

Pizzamiglio, L., Antonucci, G., Judica, A. et al. (1992) Cognitive rehabilitation of the hemineglect disorder in chronic patients with unilateral brain damage, *Journal of Clinical and Experimental Neuropsychology*, 14: 901–23.

Pizzamiglio, L., Guariglia, C., Antonucci, G. and Zoccolotti, P. (2006) Development of a rehabilitative program for unilateral neglect, *Restorative Neurology and Neuroscience*, 24: 337–45.

Predebon, J. (1984) Age trends in the Mueller–Lyer and Ponzo illusions, *British Journal of Developmental Psychology*, 3: 99–103.

Pritchard, C.L., Dijkerman, H.C., McIntosh, R.D. and Milner, A.D. (2001) Visual and tactile size distortion in a patient with right neglect, *Neurocase*, 7: 391–6.

Ricci, R., Pia, L. and Gindri, P. (2004) Effects of illusory spatial anisometry in unilateral neglect, *Experimental Brain Research*, 154: 226–37.

Ro, T. and Rafal, R.D. (1996) Perception of geometric illusions in hemispatial neglect, *Neuropsychologia*, 34: 973–8.

Rode, G., Michel, C., Rossetti, Y., Boisson, D. and Vallar, G. (2006) Left size distortion (hyperschematia) after right brain damage, *Neurology*, 67: 1801–8.

Rode, G., Revol, P., Rossetti, Y. and Vallar, G. (2008) Left hyperschematia after right brain damage, *Neurocase*, 14: 369–77.

Savazzi, S., Posteraro, L., Veronesi, G. and Mancini, F. (2007) Rightward and leftward bisection biases in spatial neglect: two sides of the same coin? *Brain*, 130(8): 2070–84.

Vallar, G. and Baddeley, A.D. (1984) Fractionation of working memory: neuro-psychological evidence for a phonological short-term store, *Journal of Verbal Learning and Verbal Behavior*, 23: 151–61.

Vallar, G. and Daini, R. (2002) Illusions in neglect, illusions of neglect, in H.O. Karnath, A.D. Milner and G. Vallar (eds) *The Cognitive and Neural Bases of Spatial Neglect*, pp. 209–24. Oxford: Oxford University Press.

Vallar, G., Daini, R. and Antonucci, G. (2000) Processing of illusion of length in spatial hemineglect: a study of line bisection, *Neuropsychologia*, 38: 1087–97.

Vallar, G. and Perani, D. (1986) The anatomy of unilateral neglect after right hemi-sphere stroke lesions: a clinical CT/Scan correlation study in man, *Neuropsychologia*, 24: 609–22.

Vuilleumier, P. and Landis, T. (1998) Illusory contours and spatial neglect, *Neuroreport*, 9: 2481–4.

Vuilleumier, P., Valenza, N. and Landis, T. (2001) Explicit and implicit perception of illusory contours in unilateral spatial neglect: behavioural and anatomical correlates of preattentive grouping mechanisms, *Neuropsychologia*, 39: 597–610.

Watt, R. (1994) Some points about human vision and visual neglect, *Neuropsychological Rehabilitation*, 4: 213–19.

Weidner, R. and Fink, G.R. (2007) The neural mechanisms underlying the Müller–Lyer illusion and its interaction with visuospatial judgments, *Cerebral Cortex*, 17: 878–84.

Zoccolotti, P., Antonucci, G., Daini, R., Martelli, M.L. and Spinelli, D. (1997) Frame-of-reference and hierarchical-organisation effects in the rod-and-frame illusion, *Perception*, 26: 1485–94.

5 Freeing the mind: brain communication that bypasses the body

Discussion of:

Birbaumer, N., Ghanayim, N., Hinterberger, T., Iversen, I., Kotchoubey, B., Kübler, A., Perelmouter, J., Taub, E. and Flor, H. (1999)

A spelling device for the paralysed, *Nature*, 398: 297–8

Reprinted with permission from Nature Publishing Group © 1999

Foreword, background and description by Richard A.P. Roche and Seán Commins
Author's commentary by Niels Birbaumer
Peer commentary by Charles W. Anderson

Foreword

The body is the most versatile and powerful tool at the brain's disposal. Through this medium, by virtue of a cascade of electrical pulses sent from the motor cortex to the limbs, muscles and joints, our mind's influence on the outside world is exerted. The idea of bypassing this bridge between the brain and the physical environment, of controlling external objects using the power of the mind alone, has traditionally been the stuff of science fiction. But in recent years, through the application of advanced technology and neuroscience research, this once seemingly impossible dream is being put to use in helping some of medicine's most isolated patients, those who have lost control of their bodies, to communicate.

Introduction

There are many types of prison. Most of them share common features – high walls, barred windows, remote locations, watchful guards. The one key characteristic that all prisons must share is the fact that they are designed to prevent escape, to keep the inmates inside. The idea of incarceration, the removal of one's freedom, is one that strikes deep at the core of what we feel it means to be human. Perhaps this is one reason for the enduring popularity of stories on the topic, from Alexandre Dumas's *Count of Monte Cristo* to Clint Eastwood's *Escape from Alcatraz* and Stephen King's *Shawshank Redemption*. But when the prison in question is one's own body, when a person becomes incarcerated within the walls of his or her own skin, a very different set of challenges can arise.

A number of medical conditions can result in large-scale physical paralysis. These include hemiplegia, the inability to control or move an arm or leg following a stroke, and quadriplegia/tetraplegia (paralysis affecting all four limbs). Typically, these disorders involve damage to some part of the circuit connecting the motor areas of the brain (supplementary motor, pre-motor and motor cortices) to the torso and limbs via the spinal cord. Disruption of this pathway means that the message to move a particular body part never arrives at its intended destination, and that limb will lie still, as if dead. While all cases of such paralysis or plegia are severely debilitating, in most cases some movement control is retained. For example, following spinal cord injury sustained in a show jumping accident, actor Christopher Reeve retained control over the muscles of his head and face until his death in 2004 and physicist Stephen Hawking, paralysed due to motor neuron disease has motor control of his eye and cheek muscles, allowing him to operate his computerized voice-box to communicate. Yet inmates such as these, severely impaired though they undoubtedly are, must be considered relatively lucky compared to another set of prisoners in this penitentiary of the body. There exists a small group of people – typically one or two in every 100,000 – who suffer from the rare conditions of amyotrophic lateral sclerosis (ALS) or total locked-in syndrome. For such patients, virtually no motor control is spared – they are truly trapped ('locked in', as the evocative title suggests) within an immobile shell, unable to move any part of their body, completely deprived of any means of communication. For them, the sentence is life in solitary confinement.

In his poignant and memorable book *The Diving Bell and the Butterfly*, former Parisian magazine editor Jean-Dominique Bauby relates his experience of having an almost classic case of total locked-in syndrome – 'almost' because his stroke left him with control over his left eyelid. Though meagre, this one remnant of physical control allowed Bauby, using a painstaking and carefully derived system involving blinks, to dictate the contents of his account. In it, he conveys the almost unimaginable feeling of being trapped within his own body, unable to move or stretch, blink or cough, swallow or yawn, scream or smile, laugh or weep. All too able to think and feel, hear and see, fear and dream, smell and imagine, remember and despair. He conjures the sense of being sealed in a tiny room with windows of one-way glass and sounds coming in, but soundproofed on the inside to allow no noise out. Yet most ALS/locked-in patients are not even so lucky as Bauby; he at least was gifted a tiny hole in the wall of his cell, enough to let a small signal out, a flicker, a small indication of intent, like Morse code. For the majority of these rare patients, even this is beyond the ability of their inert bodies. It seemed that they were destined to remain forever cut off and silent within the walls of bone and skin.

In recent years, however, these patients have been provided with a small chink of light in the darkness. The source of this reprieve originated, somewhat unexpectedly, from within – the endless and noisy chatter of ten billion neurons that continue their minute and hectic activity inside their catatonic home. Within the last decade, researchers began to use the frantic hum of these cell populations to enable locked-in patients to communicate with those around them. By recording the massed electrical signals of firing brain cells – the electroencephalogram (EEG) – from the scalp with metal electrodes, the *thought-translation device* (an example of a brain-computer interface, or BCI) converts this electrical signal into a command that can be used to move a cursor on a screen. Once this can be achieved, then the patient has the ability to direct the cursor to a particular letter, making it possible to (eventually) generate a message to the outside world from the person trapped within. In fact, one of the ironies associated with total paralysis is that the EEG signal obtained from immobile patients tend to be free of muscle artefacts or electrical 'noise' from movements, and so far cleaner than those from a normal participant – any human electrophysiologist will readily discuss at length the problems associated with extracting a clean EEG signal from a participant who will not sit still.

But obtaining the EEG signal from the patient's brain is only the first stage of a slow and frustrating process in which they must learn how to modulate their own brain activity in order to move the cursor on the screen. The patient must somehow find a way to effectively change the pitch of the clamour of brain cells, or make them sing the same song, so that some *change* can be detected by the device that monitors these cells firing from outside. It is this change in the EEG signal that will allow the thought-translation device to send the signal that will move the cursor on the screen. This task must be daunting for any patient – asking them to move a dot on a computer screen by changing what their brain is doing. Some tactics appear to include imagining they are running, or carrying out mental arithmetic, or simply relaxing. The success of the strategy will depend somewhat on the particular aspect of the EEG signal that is being used to detect a change, as there are several (elaborated in the next section).

But whatever technique they choose to use, the patient will face a long and frustrating training period, typically consisting of several hundred training sessions, in which they will become more skilled at modulating their brain activity in order to exert control over the on-screen cursor. And even when they have achieved this level of proficiency, the effect will not be the same as having the ability to whisk a mouse back and forth, guiding the cursor to any chosen area of the screen – they will simply be able to cause the cursor to very slowly move a small distance up or down. While this may seem like scant reward for such an arduous and time-consuming investment, it is the key to allowing the patient to communicate with the world from which they have been exiled. And it is worth remembering that most prison breaks involve years, if not decades, of tedious and gradual labour. Through the use of such brain-computer interfaces, it has become possible for such patients, some of the most cruelly imprisoned and profoundly isolated in medical science, to pass a note or two from the confines of their cell to the people on the outside.

Background and description of the study

Two locked-in patients suffering from amyotrophic lateral sclerosis (ALS) participated in this study. At the time of the study both patients were at an advanced stage of the disease having been fed and artificially respirated for four years. Unfortunately, both were unable to voluntarily control their muscle movements and therefore were unable to use any form of muscle-driven communication device. Many studies, however, have demonstrated that humans can learn to control components of their EEG waveforms without the need of muscle control (e.g. Birbaumer et al., 1990). One EEG component that humans can reliably control is the slow cortical potential (SCP) amplitude centred at the top of the scalp (Cz position of the international 10–20 system). Although other EEG components have been used (e.g. alpha-rhythm), employing the SCP waveform offers many advantages over others including the fact that it can be reliably produced in every person, it is highly individualistic and the underlying neurophysiology is better understood compared to other EEG features.

The patients in the current study were trained to produce changes in their SCPs that would last between two and four seconds. The procedure required the patients to view a PC screen at a distance of approximately 140 cm on which two goals (rectangles) and a small movable object (ball) were displayed (see Figure 5.1). Each trial consisted of a two-second phase during which a low tone was sounded that was then followed by a high tone (referred to as the active phase), and a two-second phase in which the high pitch tone was followed by the low tone (referred to as the baseline phase). The centred ball was only mobile in the active phase during which each patient was required to move the ball to a targeted rectangle. The goal rectangle was highlighted on the screen (see Figure 5.1) to indicate the desired direction of movement. Any change in SCP amplitude was indicated by the movement of the ball away from the centre position and towards the target. Therefore the ball's movement provided the patient with visual feedback on their own SCP. The more positive the waveform, the more the ball moved away from the centre towards the lower rectangle; while the more negative the potential, the greater the movement towards the upper goal.

Initially, both patients were required to produce a 5 µV change in the SCP; this response criterion was progressively increased to 8 µV. Both patients were better able to produce positive changes compared to negative changes, so training continued using positive changes only. As soon as the patients were reliably able to produce a consistent positive SCP change (getting at least 75 per cent correct responses lasting for a minimum of 500 ms at 8 µV), patients were then able to operate the spelling device. The first patient (Subject A: Figure 5.2, upper panel) achieved this

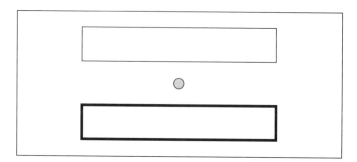

Figure 5.1 Example of display screen used in brain-computer interface with the lower goal rectangle highlighted as the target. The central grey ball will move down when the patient's slow cortical potential (SCP) of the EEG signal becomes more positive.

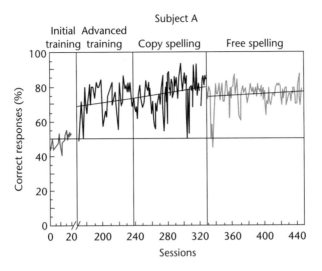

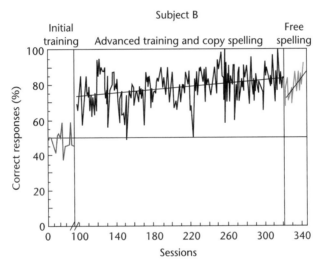

Figure 5.2 Response accuracy of subjects using the new spelling device. Subject A began with feedback training of SCP amplitude (initial and advanced training; 71.3% correct selections, 75.0% correct rejections, based on go-back responses), proceeded to copy spelling (copying of letters and then words; 78.7%, 75.3%) and finally to free spelling (self-selected letters; 66.4%, 82.9%). Subject B began with initial training, then switched to a combination of advanced training (77.5%, 68.8%) and copy spelling (77.5%, 67.6%) and finally to free spelling (86.2%, 73.7%).

Source: Reprinted with permission from Nature Publishing Group: *Nature* (Birbaumer et al., 1999) © (1999).

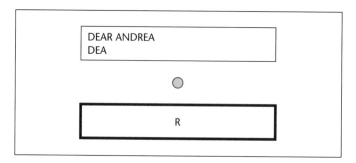

Figure 5.3 Example screen display from the training procedure for brain-computer interface. In the upper rectangle, the top line displays the sentence fragment to be copied by the patient. The second line shows letters already selected. Candidate letters are presented in the lower rectangle, which can be selected or rejected by the patient using the change in SCP signal.

after 327 sessions, and the second (Subject B: Figure 5.2, lower panel) reached this after 288 sessions.

As part of the advanced training, patients also had to copy letters and words. This was achieved by controlling a cursor in a similar fashion to that described above. On the display screen there were again two rectangles. The required words or letters that the patient was requested to spell out appeared in the top rectangle (Figure 5.3, top rectangle first line). The letters/words already selected by the patient also appeared in the top rectangle, but along the second line. The set of letters for selection was displayed in the bottom rectangle. In Figure 5.3, for example, the patient has already spelt DEA from the requested phrase DEAR ANDREA. The patient has to select the letter 'R' next by moving the ball into the bottom goal; this is again achieved by producing a large positive change in their SCP. If the character that appears in the lower triangle is not the required letter, the patient tries to keep the ball away from the goal area.

Having reached the criterion for this phase of training, patients were then given a third phase in which they could select their own letters. For this spelling program, the alphabet was split into two. The first half of the alphabet was displayed on the screen for between four and six seconds and this was followed immediately by a four-to-six-second display of the second half of the alphabet. The patient modulated their SCP for the screen that contained their required letter (see Figure 5.4). Once this was selected, the remaining letters were again split into two. The patient selected the screen containing the targeted letter by generating another positive-going SCP. This continued until a single letter was selected. This single letter was then displayed in the box at the top of the screen and the process started again with the full alphabet.

If two successive screens appeared in which no letter set was selected, a 'Go back' option was then displayed. This allowed the patient to go back to the preceding level of letter sets. If the patient was at the first level, selecting the 'Go back' function

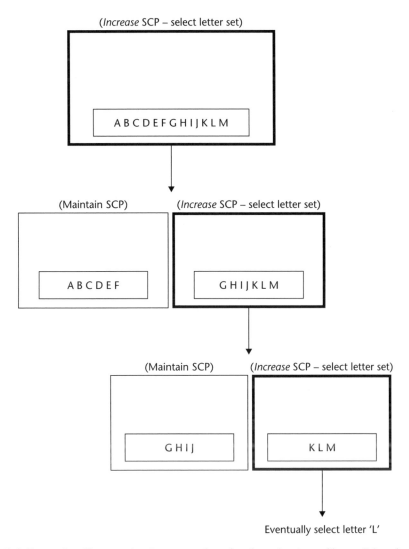

Figure 5.4 Example of letter selection procedure for the selection of letter 'L' – when the desired half of the alphabet is presented on screen, the participant modulates SCP to select. The selected letter set is then halved and each half is presented separately again. For the undesired half, the patient maintains unchanged SCP for 4–6 seconds, after which time the screen moves on to the next half of the letter set. This process is repeated until only one letter remains.

allowed the patient to erase the last symbol in the text field at the top of the screen. From this description, it is clear that this gradual selection of letters is very time consuming, working out at approximately two characters per minute. Subject A, for example, took 16 hours to write the following message.

LIEBER HERR BIRBAUMER,

HOFFENTLICH KOMMEN SIE MICH BESUCHEN, WENN DIESERBRIEF
SIE ERREICHT HAT. ICH DANKE IHNEN UND IHREM TEAM
UND BESONDERS FRAU KUBLER SEHR HERZLICH, DENN SIE
ALLE HABEN MICH ZUM ABC SCHUTZEN GEMACHT, DER OFT
DIE RICHTIGEN BUCHSTABEN TRIFFT. FRAU KUBLER IST
EINEMOTIVATIONSKUNSTLERIN.

OHNE SIE WARE DIESER BRIEF NICHTZUSTANDE
GEKOMMEN. ER MUSS GEFEIERT WERDEN. DAZU MOCHTE
ICH SIE UND IHR TEAM HERZLICH EINLADEN.
EINE GELEGENHEIT FINDET SICH HOFFENTLICH BALD.

MIT BESTEN GRUSSEN
IHR

HANS-PETER SALZMANN

Dear Mr Birbaumer,

Hopefully you will come to visit me when this letter has reached you. I thank you and your team – particularly Mrs Kübler – very much, because you all have turned me into a first class speller, who rarely misses a letter. Mrs Kübler is a motivational wizard. Without her this letter would not exist. This calls for a celebration, to which I would like to warmly invite you and your team. I hope that an opportunity will arise soon.

With best regards,

Yours truly,

Hans-Peter Salzmann.

Author commentary by Niels Birbaumer

The origin of the study in *Nature* can be traced back to the 1960s and 1970s of the past century. As a student of physiological psychology at the University of Vienna, I came across some papers by Neal E. Mille, a physiological psychologist at Rockefeller University in New York City. He claimed that voluntary control of autonomic functions is possible through operant conditioning of physiological responses (Miller, 1969). Neal's dictum was unheard before and questioned two classic assumptions: in physiology, that the autonomic nervous system is 'autonomous', independent of voluntary-motor control; in psychology that operant Skinnerian conditioning is reserved for motor responses, while classical Pavlovian conditioning is reserved for autonomic, visceral systems (see Mazur, 2004 for a review). To prove his point, Neal – who later became a friend and fatherly mentor after I visited his lab around 1971 – curarized rats for long time periods and kept them alive in the completely paralysed state for weeks and months. His students trained the rats to increase and decrease several bodily visceral responses such as heart rate, rhenal blood flow, skin temperature and other variables by rewarding them for response changes with intracranial 'pleasure' stimulation of the dopaminergic brain systems.

Curarization eliminated all possible motor mediation of the learned 'voluntary' visceral responses, proving the point: operant-voluntary control of visceral and cortical variables is possible. At the same time, the first reports of biofeedback of brain waves, particularly alpha waves, appeared (Kamiya, 1971). A graduate student and behaviorally oriented psychologist like myself was galvanized by these results: many intractable diseases seem to be accessible and treatable using operant learning principles! A few years later it turned out to be impossible to replicate those experiments (Dworkin and Miller, 1986) and brain wave biofeedback produced many meaningless clinical 'successes' in uncontrolled studies. The field died away but my 'spiritual galvanization' from that period remained and still holds until today, 40 years later: failure to replicate Neal's experiments and the difficulties with operant learning of visceral functions did not change my belief that even if the peripheral muscular system is blocked, the cortical and subcortical motor systems may affect the central autonomic system centres and through this route, operant-voluntary control of autonomic functions would be possible.

I tried to prove my point in many experiments with healthy and clinical populations (see Birbaumer et al., 1990; Birbaumer, 2006 for review) and at the same time we tried successfully to establish brainwave control as a useful clinical treatment for severe neurological disorders such as chronic pain (Flor and Birbaumer, 2000) and focal epilepsies (Kotchoubey et al., 2001).

The positive therapeutic results with drug-resistant epilepsies motivated me to use SCPs as the main target variable in completely paralysed people: these potentials had a lasting fascination since my student days; negative SCPs precede volition, and mobilize the brain for motor, cognitive and emotional responding (see Birbaumer et al., 1990). In 20 years of research we uncovered some of the neurophysiological mechanisms behind SCPs and published a comprehensive book on the subject (Rockstroh et al., 1989). After the first attempts to train paralysed patients with amyotrophic lateral sclerosis to use their SCP 'at will', it became obvious that my students could not cope with the extended training times of these very ill patients; they revolted because they needed publishable results for their theses. The grant agencies would not give money for research on a few patients only resulting in publications after many years. I was close to giving up, but 'Fortuna', the great goddess of the desperate, helped. The Deutsche Forschungsgemeinschaft (DFG; the German NIH) awarded me a five-year grant, the highest research award in Germany: €3 million without any conditions, reports, papers, and so on, the Leibniz award. Obviously, some reviewers found it worthwhile to continue my *idée fixe* of brain control through operant conditioning. After five years of training, attempts, experiments, ups and downs, the first success, a study with two locked-in patients, was published in that short *Nature* report.

These two, and the forty other ALS patients we trained over the course of the following years, finally proved that operant control of autonomous and brain functions is possible without motor mediation. Thirty-five of the patients and the two reported in the *Nature* paper had some residual motor control from time to time, mostly of the eye muscles. Their successful brain control could have been aided by peripheral motor 'mediation'; therefore the results do not prove the hypothesis of operant control of autonomic and brain function. Those eight ALS patients from our sample who are in a completely locked-in state did not succeed in brain control and communication, reflecting the replication problems encountered in Neal Miller's lab: at a physiological level the locked-in patient resembles the curarized animal in the lab (see Kübler and Birbaumer, 2008).

What can we do to solve this basic science problem and the clinical consequences? I formulated the 'extinction of goal-directed thinking' hypothesis to explain the failure of voluntary brain control in complete paralysis (see Birbaumer and Cohen, 2007; Birbaumer et al., 2008): The locked-in state deprives the patient of all contingent consequences for voluntary thoughts ('wishes') and behaviour, leading to selective extinction of all cognitive responses associated with goal-directed motor-voluntary control. To regain control of these thoughts, and their associated EEG-based brain signatures (or other brain signals), we developed a new research programme for the next years:

1 Implantation of electrodes in the brain of patients to improve signal-to-noise ratio.
2 Implement vascular brain changes such as BOLD in fMRI and near infrared spectroscopy (NIRS) instead of/together with neuroelectric signals, because self-control of brain metabolic signals is easier and faster, probably because the vascular system of the brain provides accurate feedback about its changes during learning, while neuroelectric changes are difficult to detect. First results are rewarding (Sitaram et al., 2007; Caria et al., 2007).
3 Automatization of brain training long before patients enter the completely locked-in state and assist the transfer from locked-in to completely locked-in state.
4 Include classical conditioning of 'yes' and 'no' brain responses in the paradigms.
5 Use chronic stroke and movement restoration in hemiplegic patients as a model system to retrain lost motor function with BCI, and combine it with behavioural treatment in patients with complete loss of voluntary function of one isolated brain system or the efferent pathways only. First results are very promising (Buch et al., 2008).

Acknowledgements: DFG, BMBF (Bernstein), IRCCS Ospedale San Camillo.

Peer commentary by Charles Anderson

In 1992, Jorge Aunon introduced me to the notion that patterns in EEG signals might provide a new mode of communication for patients who have no or severely limited muscle control. At that time, Keirn and Aunon (1990) showed that EEG from subjects performing several mental tasks, such as mental multiplication and imaginary rotation of geometric objects, contained patterns related to the mental task being performed. This suggested that a person could, for example, answer 'yes' or 'no' to a question by doing one or the other mental task.

In my initial work in this area, I eagerly applied some of the latest classification methods from the machine learning field to the problem of EEG pattern classification (Anderson et al., 1994, 1995). While these methods were successful for the limited data that were available, it was difficult to analyse the resulting classifiers. This drove our subsequent efforts to use simpler classifiers which, surprisingly, classified EEG data as well as the more complex methods. Thus, we were reminded of the modelling dictum that we had ignored, 'The simplest model is often the best'.

Similar conclusions were reached by researchers in labs such as those in Austria,[1] Germany[2] and Switzerland.[3] The key to a successful brain-computer interface (BCI) seems to be the use of a known pattern in EEG related to particular mental tasks. These groups and others capitalized on the known mu-rhythm, a suppression of EEG in the 8 to 12 Hz range over motor cortex contralateral to hand, arm or leg movement. This mu-rhythm was found to be present even for imagined movements, thus driving the recent work in BCIs. It was hoped that such patterns could be detected in short windows of time – less than one second – leading to fast BCIs. Unfortunately, it appears that these patterns are not continuously present and cannot be detected in all subjects. I wondered if subjects could be trained to produce consistent and more easily detected patterns.

It was at this time that I first heard of Niels Birbaumer's work, at the first workshop on the subject entitled Brain-computer Interface (BCI) Technology: Theory and Practice, at Rensselaerville Institute, New York, June, 1999. Here was someone whose lab had been conducting experiments to address these issues for years! They trained subjects through biofeedback to learn to control the SCP, a signal that can be detected quite reliably over a matter of several seconds from subjects who have undergone training. Their population of subjects even includes patients with ALS. SCPs were initially studied by Birbaumer as a means for decreasing the chances of a seizure in patients with epilepsy (Birbaumer, 1999). He quickly adapted his method into one of the most reliable approaches to BCI.

Seeing the successful use of BCIs achieved by Birbaumer's subjects convinced me that practical BCI systems are realizable much sooner than I had thought. This changed my research goals; I started developing an inexpensive, on-line BCI system with the purpose of adapting it for use by a number of patients.

In our current work, we still strive for fast decision-making using more complex patterns over multiple electrodes, but we remain grounded by Birbaumer's work. The methodology and research directions developed by him remind us that the benefit to the patient must come first. His influence leads us to focus on questions such as: how easy is it for the patient to learn to use, how easy is it to train the computer, and how reliable is the system from the user's perspective? The quality of any BCI system must be measured by the usability for the patient, and not just by higher classification accuracy on previously collected data. Investigators in the BCI research field are not immune to the temptation of staying in the research labs and publishing papers. Birbaumer and his colleagues have led the way towards the benefits that are only realizable when someone has the courage to take new technology out of the lab and into people's homes to directly enrich their lives.

Notes

1 Laboratory of brain-computer interfaces, Institute for Knowledge Discovery, Graz University of Technology, Austria: www.bci.tugraz.at
2 Berlin brain-computer interface, intelligent data analysis group, Frounhofer First Institute, Germany: www.ida.first.fraunhofer.de/bbci/index_en.html
3 Brain machine interfaces, Idiap, Switzerland: www.im2.ch/research/im2-projects/im2bmi

References

Anderson, C.W., Devulapalli, S. and Stolz, E.A. (1994) EEG as a means of communication: preliminary experiments in EEG analysis using neural networks. Proceedings of ASSETS'94, the First International ACM/SIGCAPH Conference on Assistive Technologies, pp. 141–7, New York: ACM Press.

Anderson, C.W., Devulapalli, S. and Stolz, E.A. (1995) Determining mental state from EEG signals using neural networks, *Scientific Programming*, 4(3): 171–83.

Birbaumer, N. (1999) Slow cortical potentials: plasticity, operant control, and behavioral effects, *Neuroscientist*, 5(2): 74–8.

Birbaumer, N. (2006) Breaking the silence: brain-computer-interfaces (BCI) for communication and motor control, *Psychophysiology*, 43: 517–32.

Birbaumer, N. and Cohen, L. (2007) Brain-computer-interfaces (BCI): communication and restoration of movement in paralysis, *The Journal of Physiology*, 579(3): 621–36.

Birbaumer, N., Elbert, T., Canavan, A. and Rockstroh, B. (1990) Slow potentials of the cerebral cortex and behavior, *Physiological Reviews*, 70: 1–41.

Birbaumer, N., Ramos Murguialday, A. and Cohen, L. (2008) Brain-computer interface in paralysis, *Current Opinion in Neurology*, 21(6): 634–8.

Buch, E., Weber, C., Cohen, L.G., Braun, C. et al. (2008) Think to move: a neuromagnetic brain-computer interface (BCI) system for chronic stroke, *Stroke*, 39: 910–17.

Caria, A., Veit, R., Sitaram, R., Lotze, M., Weiskopf, N., Grodd, W. and Birbaumer, N. (2007) Regulation of anterior insular cortex activity using real-time fMRI, *NeuroImage*, 35: 1238–46.

Dworkin, B.R. and Miller, N.E. (1986) Failure to replicate visceral learning in the acute curarized rat preparation, *Behavioral Neuroscience*, 100: 299–314.

Flor, H. and Birbaumer, N. (2000) Phantom limb pain: cortical plasticity and novel therapeutic approaches, *Current Opinion in Anaesthesiology*, 13: 561–4.

Kamiya, J. (ed.) (1971) *Biofeedback and Self-control: An Aldine Reader on the Regulation of Bodily Processes and Consciousness*. Chicago, IL: Aldine.

Keirn, Z.A. and Aunon, J.I. (1990) A new mode of communication between man and his surroundings, *IEEE Transactions on Biomedical Engineering*, 37(12): 1209–14.

Kotchoubey, B., Strehl, U., Uhlmann, C. et al. (2001) Modification of slow cortical potentials in patients with refractory epilepsy: a controlled outcome study, *Epilepsia*, 42(3): 406–16.

Kübler, A. and Birbaumer, N. (2008) Brain-computer interfaces and communication in paralysis: extinction of goal directed thinking in completely paralysed patients? *Clinical Neurophysiology*, 119(11): 2658–66.

Mazur, J. (2004) *Learning and Behavior*. Upper Saddle River, NJ: Prentice Hall.

Miller, N. (1969) Learning of visceral and glandular responses, *Science*, 163: 434–45.

Rockstroh, B., Elbert, T., Canavan, A., Lutzenberger, W. and Birbaumer, N. (1989) *Slow Cortical Potentials and Behaviour*, 2nd edn. Baltimore, MA: Urban & Schwarzenberg.

Sitaram, R., Zhang, H., Guan, C. et al. (2007) Temporal classification of multi-channel near-infrared spectroscopy signals of motor imagery for developing a brain-computer interface, *NeuroImage*, 34: 1416–27.

6 'Seeing' emotion in blindsight: affect without awareness

Discussion of:

de Gelder, B., Vroomen, J., Pourtois, G. and Weiskrantz, L. (1999)

Non-conscious recognition of affect in the absence of striate cortex, *Neuroreport*, 10(18): 3759–63

Reprinted with permission from Lippincott, Williams and Wilkins © 1999

Foreword, background and description by Richard A.P. Roche and Seán Commins
Author's commentary by Beatrice de Gelder
Peer commentary by James Danckert

Foreword

This chapter deals with the visual system, one of the most complex and elegantly designed processing networks in the primate brain. Specifically, it explores a bizarre aspect of visual processing that may be an indication of the brain's evolutionary development, putative evidence of a second, much older visual processing pathway than the one we most heavily rely on today. Such evidence is rare, and must be inferred from the study of the paradoxical phenomenon called 'blindsight', the persistence of residual visual function despite an absence of both an intact primary visual cortex *and* any conscious awareness of stimulation. Here we consider an ingenious experiment by de Gelder et al. (1999) that seems to suggest that this phylogenetically ancient visual system may be capable of much more complex and sophisticated processing than was previously believed.

Introduction

One of the most complex activities a human brain must carry out is that of vision. To do so, sensory input from the visual world must be taken in via the eye (an impressive feat of engineering in itself, given that it effectively constitutes a camera composed entirely out of jelly and water), relayed from the retina to the brain, where the image is decomposed into its fundamental elements and later recombined to form representations of the objects that surround us. Higher-order visual areas carry out even more complex visual functions: we can identify moving objects, recognize a friend from a stranger, judge three-dimensional depth and infer someone's mood based on their facial expression. Quite aside from being a fascinating system to study in its own right, research into visual processing has revealed many organizational principles and processing features of brain function in general.

Visual information begins its journey to the visual cortex of the brain at the eyeball. Here, the image of the world is projected onto the retina, where specialized photoreceptors, rod and cone cells, are activated by light energy of different wavelengths. The rods and cones, so named for their distinctive shapes, are selective for different types of visual information – rods are concentrated at the periphery of the retina and are specialized for processing information in dark conditions, while cones are concentrated around the fovea, and are selective for processing colour and detail in bright conditions.[1] From here, processing passes down the optic nerve to a crossover point, the optic chiasm, at which location information from the left side of each visual field passes to the right hemisphere and vice versa, ensuring all visual information is processed on the opposite side of the brain. The division of labour is maintained at this level, with separate sets of cells processing colour/form information and others responsible for movement. This is a feature that will be seen throughout the system as we travel 'upstream' in the brain. The next destination as activation spreads towards the visual cortex at the posterior of the brain is the lateral geniculate nucleus (LGN), a large bundle of cells on the lateral side of the thalamus in each hemisphere that takes its name from its resemblance to a bended knee. Functional segregation is again evident as different types of information are dealt with in the upper four and lower two layers of the LGN; thence onward, via the optic radiations, to the primary visual cortex, or area V1 of the occipital lobe.

The cells in area V1 process all aspects of the visual scene, but functional segregation remains by virtue of the fact that specialized cells are organized into different anatomical areas termed 'blobs' and 'interblobs', characteristic dark and light regions that become visible when V1 tissue is stained with the enzyme cytochrome oxidase. Processing passes from here to area V2, where a similar separation is seen; this time between stripes (thick and thin) and interstripes. Again, all aspects of the scene are processed in area V2, or secondary visual cortex. From this point onward, two distinct visual processing streams appear to emerge, one which travels dorsally from V2, via areas V5 and the dorsal aspect of V3, to the parietal cortex, where information about motion and moving objects is processed. In parallel to this dorsal stream, a ventral stream projects from V2 to V4 (colour processing) and ventral V3 (colour/form) to the ventral surface of the temporal lobe where cells are selectively responsive to visual object information. Extensive cross-talk between these two streams results in the unified percept of any object within the visual field.

This description concerns what is termed the 'geniculo-striate' visual processing pathway, and research in the past 60 years from such notable figures as Hübel, Wiesel and Zeki has greatly informed our understanding of how vision is achieved by this system. But several intriguing case studies from the last century have hinted at the existence of an older processing pathway, a potential remnant of our brain's evolutionary inheritance, and one that is supported by anatomical evidence. There exists an alternate route from eye to brain; bypassing the LGN and V1/V2 areas; this older pathway moves via subcortical structures such as the pulvinar and the tectum, and projects directly to higher-order specialized visual processing areas such as V5, completely omitting both primary and secondary visual cortices of the occipital cortex. Despite being largely overlooked in the recent history of our biological evolution, this *tecto-pulvinar pathway*, the cortical 'road less travelled' for visual information, has remained in place, side by side with its younger and more sophisticated rival. Our strongest evidence that this pathway may remain functional, though figuratively overgrown and neglected, comes from the remarkable abilities of patients suffering from the rare visual condition of *blindsight*.

Discrete damage to the cortical stages of the visual system can result in a variety of symptoms and some very bizarre phenomenological experiences on the part of the patient. From small blind-spots (*scotoma*) in the visual field caused by localized damage to V1 or V2 to the loss of colour vision or motion perception due to destruction of V4 or V5, respectively, the study of such deficits following cortical insult has provided considerable insight into the nature of visual processing. Among the most common of such visual disorders is 'blindsight', a term coined by Larry Weiskrantz and first used in print in a *Lancet* article in 1974 to describe residual visual functions in patients whose primary visual cortex was absent, either through removal or damage (Sanders et al., 1974). While there had previously existed some evidence of this possibility from work with animals (for a review of blindsight in monkeys and humans, see Stoerig and Cowey, 1997), it was only after World War II, which produced a number of patients suffering from cortical blindness (who reported being blind following occipital damage, despite their visual apparatus being intact up as far as the visual cortex), that the phenomenon was observed in humans. Astonishingly, a subset of these cortically blind patients showed a high rate of accuracy when asked to 'guess' at the location or nature of visual stimuli presented to their blind visual fields. All the more curious was the fact that this good performance was achieved without any awareness of visual stimulation on their part.

Following these early reports, the patient DB (Weiskrantz et al., 1974), who would go on to become the most intensively studied blindsight patient, presented with similar visual abilities despite a lack of any conscious awareness of vision. DB had undergone surgical removal of the right occipital cortex due to the presence of a tumour, an operation which resulted in cortical blindness in DB's left visual field. As such, DB reported no visual experience of any sort in his left field, consistent with Type 1 blindsight (in contrast to Type 2, in which patients report a 'feeling' or 'know-ing' that a visual stimulus is present). Despite this lack of awareness, DB's performance when asked to guess simple visual characteristics – visual discrimination, orientation judgements, telling static from moving objects, reaching to approximate locations, and so on – was well above chance levels.

Since that time, DB and other notable blindsight patients (including GY, the patient under study in the de Gelder article with which this chapter is concerned) have been the focus of rigorous investigation, and much has been learned about the nature of such non-conscious processing. Furthermore, it now appears that this curious phenomenon is not restricted to the visual sensory modality – case studies of 'numb-sense' or 'blind touch' (Rossetti et al., 1995) and 'deaf hearing' (Michel et al., 1980; Mozaz-Garde and Cowey, 2000) have subsequently been reported and studied. But importantly, the noteworthy feature of the study to which we next turn our attention is the fact that, rather than testing very basic visual functions such as discrimination and motion detection, de Gelder and colleagues set out to investigate whether a higher-order, complex and highly sophisticated function such as emotional recognition based on facial expression might be spared in the blindsight patient GY.

Background and description of the study

A single patient (GY) suffering from blindsight took part as a participant in this study. GY, a 43-year-old man (at the time of study), suffered damage to his left occipital cortex in a car accident when he was 8 years of age. As a result of the accident he has right field blindness. Previous behavioural testing (Weiskrantz et al., 1998) demonstrated GY as having blindsight, with a residual visual capacity to detect, localize and discriminate stimuli in his blind hemifield. As most previous studies conducted with blindsight patients have typically examined perception of elementary visual information such as discrimination of shapes, colour, perception of movement and direction of movement, the authors wished, in this study, to examine whether higher level and more complex visual stimuli could also be detected. Specifically, de Gelder et al. wished to determine whether GY could discriminate between different facial emotions, and if so whether this discrimination could be done unconsciously. In addition, the authors wished to determine whether any neural correlates of this discrimination could be detected in GY's blind field using ERP analysis.

In an initial experiment, the authors presented eight blocks of stimulus pairs to GY's blind field and intact field. The stimulus pairs consisted of short video clips of a female face pronouncing the same sentence with a happy or sad facial expression, an angry or sad facial expression, and an angry or fearful facial expression. The stimulus pairs were presented either randomly to both visual fields or as a block of trials to either field. GY's task was to guess the facial expression presented to his blind field. When the stimuli were presented to his intact left visual field, GY's performance was almost flawless. Alternatively, when asked to say what he saw when the stimuli were presented to his blind field, GY responded that he observed the offset and onset of a white flash, but never consciously observed a face or a moving stimulus. However, he guessed correctly on 66 per cent of the trials presented to his blind right visual field (220/333 trials). Table 6.1 gives a breakdown of the number of correct responses given by GY for the

Table 6.1 Covert recognition of facial expressions

Stimulating pair	Image size	L/R presentation	Correct	p
Happy/fearful	Small	Randomized	22/27	<0.001
Happy/fearful	Large	Randomized	18/28	NS
Happy/fearful	Small	Blocked	37/58	<0.05
Happy/fearful	Large	Blocked	37/58	<0.05
Angry/sad	Small	Randomized	15/27	NS
Angry/sad	Small	Blocked	39/54	<0.01
Angry/fearful	Small	Randomized	15/27	NS
Angry/fearful	Small	Blocked	37/56	<0.05

Table 6.2 Confusion matrix of GY's response to happy, sad, angry or fearful videos

Video	Response			
	Happy	Sad	Angry	Fearful
Happy	27	2	6	1
Sad	1	24	5	6
Angry	3	11	13	9
Fearful	2	12	6	15

stimulus pairs presented to his blind visual field according to the various conditions of the experiment (whether the different pairs were presented to the visual field randomly or as a block of trials, and whether the image presentation was large or small). As observed from the final column, in the majority of conditions, GY responded with significantly greater accuracy than would be expected if he responded solely based on chance.

In the second experiment, instead of allowing GY to guess the facial expressions of pairs of stimuli, the authors requested GY to guess the presented expression given the choice of four emotions (happy, sad, angry, fearful), thereby making the task slightly harder. The presentations were given in two blocks and were made to the blind right visual field only. On the first block, GY correctly guessed the facial expression on 38 out of 72 trials (each of the four emotions was presented 18 times). This 52 per cent correct response rate was found to be significantly higher than chance level (at 25 per cent). In the second block of presentations, GY improved slightly, guessing correctly on 41 out of 72 trials (57 per cent correct response rate). Table 6.2 shows the breakdown of responses that GY made to each of the four presented video clips. This table also demonstrates that GY was better at recognizing the happy and sad than the angry and fearful videos. For example, if the video segment showed a happy expression, GY correctly labelled this as happy in 27 out of 36 trials, and only guessed this clip as sad, angry or fearful in 2, 6 and 1 trials, respectively. By contrast, if the video clip presented a fearful expression, GY labelled this clip as fearful in 15 trials out of 36, and as sad in 12 trials out of 36.

In the third experiment, the authors tested whether GY would be able to identify facial emotions better if they were presented in a moving video rather than as picture stills. Similar to the second experiment, the stimuli were presented to GY's blind field. GY was instructed to guess the emotion given the choice of either a happy or fearful face. In addition, GY's performance was tested with video fragments and still photographs that were either upright or inverted. Table 6.3 demonstrates that GY guessed the emotion correctly in 19 out of 27 presentations of still upright photographs (significantly better than chance levels). He also guessed the correct emotion in 20 out of 28 dynamic (moving video) upright clips presented randomly and in 51 out of 56 trials of upright video clips presented in blocked fashion (both significantly above chance levels). These results would suggest that movement plays an important role in allowing GY to perceive and detect emotion.

In the final experiment, which was conducted a few months after the first three, the authors again tested GY on pairs of emotions (happy/sad, angry/fearful) presented to

Table 6.3 Perceiving facial expressions or discriminating movement

Stimulus	Orientation	Presentation	Correct	p
Dynamic	Upright	Randomized	20/28	<0.05
Still	Upright	Randomized	19/27	<0.05
Dynamic	Inverted	Randomized	18/28	NS
Still	Inverted	Randomized	16/28	NS
Dynamic	Upright	Blocked	51/56	<0.001
Still	Upright	Blocked	26/53	NS
Dynamic	Inverted	Blocked	26/56	NS
Still	Inverted	Blocked	27/54	NS

his blind field. There were two conditions in this experiment; congruent and incongruent (two blocks each). In the congruent condition, one of the response choices matched the video clip. For example, if GY was shown a happy video clip, he had to guess the emotion given the choice between happy or sad. Similarly, if given a sad video, GY had to guess whether it was displaying a happy or sad emotion. The same was true for the angry and fearful emotional pairs. However, in the incongruent condition, neither response choice mached the video clip. For example, if GY was again shown a happy video clip, he had to guess the emotion this time from a choice of angry or fearful. As with the three previous experiments, GY reported seeing a white flash with stimulus onset and offset and nothing more. His performance in the congruent conditions was better than during incongruent conditions. In the first block of congruent trials, GY correctly guessed the emotion in 44 out of 56 trials overall (78 per cent correct, significantly better than the chance level of 50 per cent). He correctly guessed the happy face in 21 out of 28 trials, and 25 out of 28 trials for the sad faces (75 per cent and 89 per cent correct, respectively; again, both were significantly greater than chance). With the angry/fearful faces, GY had more difficulty in guessing correctly (similar to the experiment shown in Table 6.2). In the first block GY was correct on only 26 out of 60 trials (43 per cent), only 15 out of 30 angry faces were guessed correctly, and 11 out of 30 fearful faces were recognized as fearful (50 per cent and 36 per cent, respectively; not significantly different from chance). However, GY improved significantly on the second block of trials, guessing 40 out of 60 correctly (67 per cent). He recognized 21 of 30 angry faces as angry, and 19 out of 30 fearful faces as fearful (70 per cent and 63 per cent, respectively; this time significantly better than chance). In the incongruent conditions, when GY was shown either an angry or fearful video, he tended to guess sad over happy. In addition, when shown either a happy or sad video, GY tended to guess fear rather than anger (see Table 6.4).

Finally, event-related brain potentials (ERPs) were recorded from GY in response to static neutral, happy or fearful faces presented randomly to either his intact left or blind right visual field. GY was required to guess the gender of these faces. GY correctly recognized the gender 92.8 per cent of times when the faces were presented to his intact field. When presented to his blind field, GY guessed correctly in 51.4 per cent of trials. His difficulty with static images confirms the results presented in the experiment in Table 6.3. Figure 6.1 shows grand average visual ERPs (combined for both happy and

Table 6.4 GY's labelling of the videos with congruent and incongruent ideas

Video		Response	
Angry/fearful videos			
		Happy	Sad
Angry		24	36
Fearful		24	36
Happy/sad videos			
		Fear	Angry
Happy		33	27
Sad		32	28

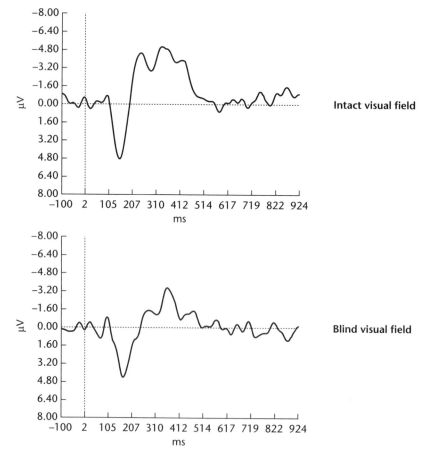

Figure 6.1 Grand average for visual ERPs recorded at Oz site for happy and fearful faces (combined) presented to the intact (top) and blind (bottom) visual fields. Negativity is plotted upwards.

Source: Reprinted with permission from Lippincott, Williams & Wilkins: *NeuroReport* (de Gelder et al., 1999), © (1999).

fearful faces) recorded over the occipital Oz site. Visual stimulation in the intact visual field (Figure 6.1, top) revealed a positive deflection peaking at 148.62 ms with an amplitude of 4.83 μV. This was followed by a negative deflection peaking with an amplitude of −4.50 μV occurring at 240.02 ms. Visual presentation in GY's blind field evoked a similar positive deflection peaking at 4.44 μV occurring at 164.04 ms, followed by smaller negative component (−1.50 μV) occurring at 276 ms (see Figure 6.1). These electrophysiological results clearly demonstrate visually evoked activity when material is presented to the blind field in the absence of conscious recognition of the presented stimuli.

Author commentary by Beatrice de Gelder

Affective blindsight refers to the residual visual ability of patients with damage to the primary visual cortex (V1, striate cortex) to react reliably to the emotional valence of stimuli presented to their blind visual fields, while remaining unable to report the presence and properties of these stimuli. To the extent that non-conscious vision can be created by experimental techniques in normally-seeing individuals, their residual abilities are also referred to as affective blindsight when it concerns emotional stimuli.

The first report that a patient with blindsight could discriminate (with a reliability exceeding chance level) the emotion of stimuli he could not consciously perceive was published by de Gelder and co-workers in 1999 (de Gelder et al., 1999). The study was conducted on the well-known patient GY with blindness in his right visual field following damage to the left occipital lobe, and consisted of four different experiments in which short video fragments and still images showing different facial expressions were used as stimuli. Common to all experiments was the use of direct methodologies requiring the patient to 'guess' (in various forced-choice conditions) the emotion conveyed by stimuli he remained unaware of. At that time, there was initial evidence from animal and human studies that subcortical structures (like the amygdala in the medial temporal lobe) were able to react to emotionally laden stimuli in the environment and to initiate appropriate responses towards them even before a detailed perceptual analysis was provided by primary sensory cortices (LeDoux, 1996; Morris et al., 1998; Whalen et al., 1998).

However, until recently investigation of non-conscious perception in blindsight had focused predominantly on basic psychophysical properties such as discrimination of simple shapes, gratings, movement or colour (Weiskrantz et al., 1974; Weiskrantz, 1986, 2004). The finding that blindsight subjects can discriminate something as subtle as facial expressions without the contribution of primary visual cortex is, however, less puzzling when viewed against a broader biological context. Indeed, behavioural manifestations of emotion conveyed by the face or by whatever other means (including vocalizations and body language) have a high communicative function in many species (Darwin, 1872; Hatfield et al., 1994; de Gelder, 2006).

The initial investigations of affective blindsight in my lab were not really planned. A different set of experiments had been carefully prepared by me and my colleagues, and only at the last minute did we decide to take a risk with running the emotion experiments that were available but had so far been undertaken for a very different purpose. The motivation for bringing the blindsight patient to the lab (but not for doing the emotion experiments) was this: a recurrent theme in experiments on audiovisual integration and a matter of great concern for the theories is whether or not the obtained crossmodal bias effects are taking place online during the perceptual process itself or originate in the postperceptual judgment that is required from the study participant. My colleague Paul Bertelson and I had already discussed this question in detail for a couple of years. This issue had been a longstanding concern of Paul's and our discussions were actually the basis of a report in *Trends in the Cognitive Sciences* (TICS); de Gelder and Bertelson, 2003.

Rather than staying close to my previous occupation and addressing this issue in philosophical terms, I suggested to Paul that finding a population with a focal lesion that had an impact on conscious perception may be the way to go. I was in touch with Larry Weiskrantz as we were both involved in running the Society for Philosophy and Psychology, so I asked him whether it would be possible to test his famous blindsight patient GY. This appeared feasible and we prepared the experiment, which also involved Jean Vroomen (who had completed his PhD thesis with me on audiovisual speech perception). The goal, obviously, was to measure whether the visual stimuli that were not consciously perceived (due to the lesion that rendered GY blind in his right hemifield) would exert a bias on GY's auditory percept. If this was found to be the case, it would provide evidence for crossmodal bias from unseen visual stimuli. As the testing sessions continued, it became clear that the sudden onset of the visual stimulus that we used, which we thought was required to run this ventriloquism experiment, simply would not do. Because of the sudden onset, GY was almost always aware of the visual stimulus and we did not (during those sessions, at least) manage to create testing conditions where GY was unaware of the visual stimulus presented to his blind field.

Once it was clear that our efforts in this area were doomed to failure, I was in a better position to convince my friends to try the audiovisial emotion experiment. Here it was possible to modify the parameters of the visual stimulus presentation such that sudden onset and changes in luminance could be controlled This study was undertaken in a climate of humorous scepticism from the side of my two colleagues, but I was ready to take up the challenge and all of us were unhindered by any specific competence on affective cognition! Clearly, none of us knew much about that vast field of emotion research and we were not ready to jump into what we imagined to be an ocean of literature on emotions. Nevertheless, the specific issue of audiovisual integration not under conscious control fascinated all of us.

After the initial experiment was repeated a few times during the same morning, we set out to design some variants. One somewhat radical version that amused me very much given my philosophy background consisted of providing GY with two response alternatives among which he had to choose, but replacing these with choices that were not actually shown. As usual, once GY went into testing mode he responded very professionally and normally avoided any comment on the 'what' or the 'why' of the experiment. However, on this occasion there was clearly something else going on and he asked after two blocks whether we needed more data on this one. I asked what the problem was and he said that there was something that bothered him about this experiment and that he felt uneasy doing it. After these blocks some more repetitions were run using both still images and short video clips which, taken together, allowed us to conclude that there was residual vision for short video clips of facial expressions.

I mentioned this finding with great enthusiasm (and puzzlement) to two Dutch colleagues with whom I was meeting shortly after obtaining these results. They very rapidly exchanged a look of disbelief accompanied by the briefest of pitiful microfacial expressions (as beautifully described in Ekman's work, as I later learned). Larry had repeated often enough that when a fact is just that, explanations must sometimes wait; meanwhile, the fact is still a fact. But having met with some disbelief, I decided to take no risks from possibly overly sceptical friends and send this paper of ours directly to *Neuroreport* where it was accepted without further ado; it is this paper that forms the basis of this chapter.

After learning about Ray Dolan's research on unconscious recognition of facial expressions, I mentioned this result to him and it was quickly agreed that we would run a functional magnetic resonance imaging (fMRI) study. We were pleased to find that indeed there was amygdala activation triggered by the presentation of fearful facial expressions. Our study has impacted on others within this area of research and it is widely quoted, next to the subsequent brain imaging study we then did at the Functional Imaging Laboratory (FIL) in London with Ray Dolan and John Morris that followed up on our behavioural results. Most importantly, our results have been replicated in other labs with other patients (Hamm et al., 2003; Pegna et al., 2008). Moreover, a few studies have tried to create the visual perception conditions of hemianopia patients with residual blindsight in neurologically intact observers by using techniques like masking or applying transcranial magnetic stimulation (TMS) (see Chapter 2) to visual cortex (reviewed in de Gelder and Tamietto, 2007).

The finding that emotional valence of facial expressions can be reliably discriminated, even in the absence of conscious visual experience by patients with lesions to the primary visual cortex (affective blindsight), is important for a number of reasons. Whether or not attention and consciousness are prerequisites for affective perception is till a hotly debated issue. Affective blindsight in cortically blind persons presents the clearest case of non-conscious emotion perception because, when visual parameters like luminance are carefully controlled, the patients literally cannot see nor visually acknowledge the presence of a stimulus. Investigation of this condition offers a unique opportunity to understand the neuro-functional bases of emotion perception without awareness. Its importance is directly related to the fact that emotional processing in the absence of stimulus awareness is an important component of the emotional capabilities of neurologically intact individuals.

Our lab and a few others are currently running new studies to investigate in depth the neural basis of vision without striate cortex. A review of these studies in the domain of *affective blindsight* is published in *Scholarpedia* and can be accessed at www.scholarpedia.org/wiki/index.php?title=Affective_blindsight&oldid=20914

Peer commentary by James Danckert

'Blindsight' is truly one of the more fascinating neurological phenomena a cognitive neuroscientist can study. That an individual with primary occipital cortex damage can nevertheless respond at above chance levels to stimuli presented to his or her blind field seems at first to be unbelievable. The label for the phenomenon itself invokes a feeling of impossibility – how can one be blind and have sight at the same time? More than 20 years of research in numerous patients and with a multitude of techniques has nevertheless robustly demonstrated just that. Patients can reliably point to and look towards targets they report never having seen; performance for sighted field stimuli is dramatically influenced by distracting stimuli in the blind field that the patient is never aware of, and even such things as semantic priming and wavelength processing have been demonstrated for blind field stimuli. As such, blindsight raises important questions about the nature of vision, the anatomical pathways that support 'varieties' of vision in the primate brain and more interestingly, the nature of consciousness and its neural representation.

My own initial foray into blindsight started during my PhD with Dr Paul Maruff in Australia. We were interested in exploring the nature of selective mechanisms of attention and used implicit measures to examine this in two hemianopes – one with a V1 lesion and the other with a thalamic lesion. We found that the first patient showed implicit processing of blind field colour and shape information, while the patient with the thalamic lesion did not. This, and many other studies before and since, demonstrated two important aspects of blindsight: first, that basic stimulus properties such as colour and form can be processed without V1 and second, that any such processing requires that secondary pathways from the LGN of the thalamus directly to extrastriate cortex remain intact. Later, as a postdoctoral fellow with Dr Yves Rossetti in Lyon, France, we showed that localizing blind field targets by pointing to them also depended on the integrity of one of the main targets of this secondary visual pathway – the posterior parietal cortex – an intuition that Dr Weiskrantz and his colleagues had hinted at in their original work. My own approach to research on blindsight then has been to examine how the unusual (i.e. blindsight) can inform the usual (e.g. attention, visuomotor control; Danckert et al., 1998, Danckert et al., 2003).

What de Gelder and colleagues did was to extend these original studies to a domain one would not have thought possible – the recognition of facial emotions. Given the complexity of faces and the broad range of subtle changes that can imbue a face with emotion, it would seem highly unlikely that a patient who is consciously blind to these subtleties would be capable of processing them to some level. Often what we intuit about our visual experience does not match up to the reality. When we imagine looking at the face of another person and processing their emotional state, it feels as though we are consciously interpreting what we see. To ourselves we might think something like 'She looks sad today,' or 'My boss looks like he's on the war path'. But these conscious interpretations are almost certainly late-stage processes that occur *after* we have already unconsciously processed the emotional expressions of the people we are interacting with. De Gelder and colleagues conclusively demonstrate this by showing that GY was able to reliably distinguish between emotional expressions of faces he did not consciously 'see'.

The question then arises as to what conscious interpretation may add to such automatic recognition processes? Furthermore, while action-blindsight (i.e. pointing to or looking at blind field target locations) has been shown to rely on an intact posterior parietal cortex, these results imply a different target for the secondary visual pathway. Given what we know about emotional processing, the visual information conveyed to extrastriate cortex via the pulvinar in GY's case must then be conveyed to medial temporal structures such as the amygdala in order for successful recognition of emotions to arise.

Finally, what role might top-down processing have played in their results? Certainly, giving GY incongruent labels with which to make his forced choice judgements impaired his ability to recognize blind field facial emotions. There also appeared to be greater difficulty for GY in distinguishing between angry/fearful faces than happy/sad faces. This could be due to greater visual similarity in the first pair versus the second pair. What would one expect to see if a greater range or subtlety of emotions were tested? Finally, GY seemed to rely heavily on the moving components of an expression, again suggesting another part of the neural pathway – area middle temporal (MT) – that he was relying on to do this task. As with all great studies, the de Gelder study has raised as many questions as it has answered.

The de Gelder study also raises the spectre of classification of blindsight patients. In other words, are all blindsight patients the same? Weiskrantz in 1998 made an initial distinction between two subtypes of blindsight distinguished in part by whether or not the patient had a 'sense' of something happening in their blind field (Type II) or not (Type I). Yves Rossetti and I recently suggested a different classification system based on what kind of abilities the patient demonstrates (Danckert and Rossetti, 2005). We distinguished between action and attention blindsight to highlight the required output of the patient. That is, in action-blindsight the patient is required to point to, look at or grasp an object in their blind field. In attention-blindsight, forced choice paradigms of the kind used by de Gelder and colleagues are used to examine such behaviours as form discrimination. Finally, in agnosopsia, somewhat akin to Type II blindsight, anything from wavelength processing, semantic priming and perhaps recognition of facial emotions can occur. The non-specific 'sense' that some patients experience when processing blind field stimuli can accompany attention-blindsight or agnosopsia, but rarely if ever accompanies action-blindsight.

One of the key characteristics of the distinction between action- and attention-blindsight that we made was the time course over which it can be demonstrated. We reasoned that because action-blindsight required a direct motor response, it probably used secondary visual pathways that terminate in the parietal cortex and operate in a fast, automatic fashion. Therefore, you should be able to demonstrate action-blindsight in a relatively small number of trials. While some functions that we ascribed to attention-blindsight may also rely on this pathway, the means by which they are tested will determine how robust the phenomena are. For example, implicit tests of blind field processing often require the patient to respond to something they do see while a distracting stimulus is presented to their blind field. Any implicit processing of that distractor will lead to interference in processing the seen item and can again be measured in a relatively small number of trials. When it comes to using forced choice guessing, the story changes. Patients most often report seeing nothing and have to be encouraged to make a guess. Often, any demonstration of blindsight using this method takes many hundreds of trials over multiple sessions with above chance performance only becoming evident in the later sessions. It is as if the secondary pathway needs to be 'trained' to detect or discriminate more accurately what is necessarily a weaker visual input.

The de Gelder study turns this notion on its head a little by using forced choice guesses in GY with relatively few trials to show recognition of facial emotions. Not only that, but they add a direct measure of the secondary processing of blind field stimuli via ERPs. What both of these things may indicate is that the visual components of emotional expressions are robustly and automatically processed in the human brain. Secondary pathways through the pulvinar to extrastriate cortex probably carry this information more rapidly than the primary geniculostriate pathway could, thereby enabling swift recognition of the emotion of another person we are about to interact with. The implications of this for theories of emotion and social cognition are enormous and have been backed up by more recent neuroimaging studies.

To return to my own approach to blindsight research one could ask, what does the de Gelder study tell us about normal cognition? Simplistically (and there is much more to their study than one summary sentence can capture), they have demonstrated that visual information concerning facial expressions is rapidly conveyed to the extrastriate cortex, and probably beyond, in the absence of conscious visual awareness. Their combination of behavioural and ERP methods also raises the bar for blindsight research in requiring measures (e.g. ERP, fMRI, skin conductance, pupillary dilation, etc.) that can be correlated with behaviour to provide further and arguably more convincing evidence that the patient is truly and effectively processing something they simply can not see.

Note

1   This explains why, on a dark night, stars seem brighter in the periphery of vision and dimmer when one looks directly at them.

References

Danckert, J. and Rossetti, Y. (2005) Blindsight in action: what can the different sub-types of blindsight tell us about the control of visually guided actions? *Neuroscience & Biobehavioral Reviews*, 29(7): 1035–46.

Danckert, J., Maruff, P., Kinsella, G., de Graaff, S. and Currie, J. (1998) Investigating form and colour perception in blindsight using an interference task, *Neuroreport*, 9(13): 2919–25.

Danckert, J., Revol, P., Pisella, L. et al. (2003) Measuring unconscious actions in action-blindsight: exploring the kinematics of pointing movements to targets in the blind field of two patients with cortical hemianopia, *Neuropsychologia*, 41(8): 1068–81.

Darwin, C. (1872) *The Origin of Species*. London: Murray.

de Gelder B. (2006) Towards the neurobiology of emotional body language. *Nature Reviews Neuroscience*, 7(3): 242–9.

de Gelder, B. and Bertelson, P. (2003) Multisensory integration, perception and ecological validity, *Trends in Cognitive Science*, 7(10): 460–7.

de Gelder, B. and Tamietto, M. (2007) Affective blindsight, *Scholarpedia*, 2(10): 3555.

Hamm, A.O., Weike, A.I., Schupp, H.T. et al. (2003) Affective blindsight: intact fear conditioning to a visual cue in a cortically blind patient, *Brain*, 126(2): 267–75.

Hatfield, E., Cacioppo, J. and Rapson, R.L. (1994) *Emotional Contagion*. New York: Cambridge University Press.

LeDoux, J.E. (1996) *The Emotional Brain*. New York: Simon & Schuster.

Michel, F., Peronnet, F. and Schott, B.A. (1980) A case of cortical deafness: clinical and electrophysiological data, *Brain & Language*, 10(2): 367–77.

Morris, J.S., Oehman, A. and Dolan, R.J. (1998) Conscious and unconscious emotional learning in the human amygdala, *Nature*, 393: 467–70.

Mozaz-Garde, M. and Cowey, A. (2000) Deaf hearing: unacknowledged detection of auditory stimuli in a patient with cerebral deafness, *Cortex*, 36: 71–80.

Pegna, A.J., Caldara-Schnetzer, A.S. and Khateb, A. (2008) Visual search for facial expressions of emotion is less affected in simultanagnosia, *Cortex*, 44(1): 46–53.

Rossetti, Y., Rode, G. and Boisson, D. (1995) Implicit processing of somaesthetic information: a dissociation between where and how? *Neuroreport*, 6(3): 506–10.

Sanders, M.D., Warrington, E.K., Marshall, J. and Wieskrantz, L. (1974) 'Blindsight': vision in a field defect, *Lancet*, 1(7860): 707–8.

Stoerig, P. and Cowey, A. (1997) Blindsight in man and monkey, *Brain*, 120(3): 535–9.

Weiskrantz, L. (1986) Some aspects of memory functions and the temporal lobes, *Acta Neurologica Scandinavica Supplement*, 109: 69–74.

Weiskrantz, L. (2004) Roots of blindsight, *Progress in Brain Research*, 144: 229–41.

Weiskrantz, L., Warrington, E.K., Sanders, M.D. and Marshall, J. (1974) Visual capacity in the hemianopic field following a restricted occipital ablation, *Brain*, 97: 709–28.

Weiskrantz, L., Cowey, A. and Le Mare, C. (1998) Learning from the pupil: a spatial visual channel in the absence of V1 in monkey and human, *Brain*, 121: 1065–72.

Whalen, P.J., Rauch, S.L., Etcoff, N.L. et al. (1998) Masked presentations of emotional facial expressions modulate amygdala activity without explicit knowledge, *Journal of Neuroscience*, 18: 411.

7 Routes to memory: neuroplasticity in the hippocampal formation

Discussion of:

Maguire, E.A., Gadian, D.G., Johnsrude, I.S., Good, C.D., Ashburner, J., Frackowiak, R.S. and Frith, C.D. (2000)

Navigation-related structural change in the hippocampi of taxi drivers, *Proceedings of the National Academy of Science, USA*, 97(8): 4398–403

Reprinted with permission from National Academy of Science © 2000

Foreword, background and description by Richard A.P. Roche and Seán Commins
Author's commentary by Eleanor A. Maguire
Peer commentary by Shane M. O'Mara

Foreword

This chapter discusses a paper that has become a citation classic in the area of memory. It is included in this collection of studies due to its innovative approach of using a group of normal individuals whose brains have become specialized for a particular cognitive faculty due to years of training. It also demonstrates how plastic change may be possible in the brain, even for higher-order cognitive processing. Furthermore, it highlights the implications of cortical expansion for neighbouring regions, where growth of one area may result in reduced volume of its neighbour.

Introduction

Most people consider memory to be a place. The way we think about it, the language we use to articulate it, the types of analogy that are drawn to describe it – all seem to convey an image of a great repository, like a vast warehouse or library, in which our memories are kept, or 'stored'. When we want to remember something, we speak of 'retrieval' or 'recollection', as if we physically go to this storage area and search through the experiences that are stored there until we 'find' the memory that we are looking for. We speak of forgetting as the 'loss' of memory, in which we are either unable to 'find' the desired experience from the past, or we feel as though it has been removed from the store altogether. And while the computer analogy has, in recent decades, begun to infiltrate the language we use to describe memory – terms such as 'encoding' have crept in – the idea that memory is a place where events are kept remains the most accessible or convenient way for humans to conceptualize it. Perhaps it is the best way the brain has found to describe this aspect of its own function.

The process of remembering has had a long historical association with mental representations of the spatial environment. The link can be traced as far back as the ancient Greek philosophers who, in order to remember the various arguments to be presented in their oration, would envisage an imaginary temple upon whose pillars each of their theses were posted. As the orator moved mentally through the temple, he would quite literally 'arrive at' the next point to be made. More contemporary mnemonic devices similarly make use of mental spatial imagery; in the Method of Loci, the contents of a shopping list can be retained by imagining each of the grocery items in a different location as one navigates through one's own home; for example, sausages at the front door, eggs on the stairs, and so on. Clearly, memory appears to benefit from the use of a spatial framework.

Further evidence for this relationship between memory and spatial representation comes when we consider the anatomy of the brain. We have known since the late 1950s that the hippocampal formation, the seahorse-shaped structures that lie buried deep within the medial temporal lobes (MTL) of each hemisphere, play a crucial role in memory formation. The classic case study of patient HM, the 21-year-old who had his hippocampi surgically removed in 1953 in an attempt to arrest his frequent and severe epileptic seizures, revealed that an intact hippocampal formation is essential for remembering new information. Scoville and Milner (1957) report, after describing the 'frankly experimental operation', that the young HM was left with a severe antero-grade amnesia, an inability to retain any new factual information. Furthermore, HM's impairments extended to spatial memory tasks such as the memorization of sequence of turns in various types of maze (see Corkin, 2002 for a more detailed discussion of HM's spatial impairments). More evidence for the link between hippocampal structures and spatial memory comes from non-human species – small mammals and birds who must store and remember the location of food have been shown to possess hippocampi of greater volume (Lee et al., 1998), and in some species this increase in volume is closely and transiently associated with the season during which spatial memory is most pertinent (Smulders et al., 1995).

The discovery of place cells – neurons that fire selectively depending on the animal's location in a spatial environment – in the rat hippocampus (O'Keefe and Dostrovsky, 1971) and the subsequent publication of O'Keefe and Nadel's seminal 'The hippocampus as a cognitive map' in 1978 served to cement the link between hippocampal structures and spatial memory. As a result, research into spatial memory and the hippocampal formation has exploded in the past 30 years, with upwards of 2,000 articles published on the topic. Few studies in modern cognitive neuroscience have gone on to demonstrate this link as elegantly or dramatically as that of Eleanor Maguire and her colleagues in the year 2000. Her previous research had demonstrated that patients with right or left hippocampal removal were severely impaired when asked to draw a map of a route through an urban environment presented by video (Maguire et al., 1996). Drawing on this and the previous literature linking hippocampus and spatial memory, as well as emerging evidence of use-related plasticity in the human brain (see Chapter 2), the group hypothesized that repeated and extensive use of detailed spatial memories or routes might result in structural changes in the human hippocampus, changes that might be detectable by modern imaging techniques such as structural magnetic resonance imaging (MRI).

The crucial requirement for the study was to find a population of people for whom spatial navigation and recollection was a frequent and prolonged activity. The authors found the answer effectively on their doorstep – London taxi drivers are required to pass arduous and extensive training on the various routes and locations in the city that typically takes a minimum of two years to complete. This process of doing 'The Knowledge' involves the establishment of a highly sophisticated spatial representation of London, a representation on which taxi drivers need to draw on a daily basis to allow successful navigation around the city. They therefore constituted the ideal group for this study in order to address the question: would their training while 'on The Knowledge' and the day-to-day use of that spatial representation result be manifested in physical alterations in the brain regions associated with this type of memory, namely the hippocampus?

Background and description of the study

Maguire and her colleagues used 16 male London taxi drivers with an average of over 14 years of driving experience. All drivers were fully trained (having undergone 'The Knowledge') and all were generally healthy. For comparison purposes the study also used 50 males that did not drive taxis for a living. The groups were matched for both age and health status. The brains of all participants were imaged using an MRI scan and were subsequently analysed. Results from the scans indicated that there was a significant increase in grey matter volume in the taxi driver group in only two brain regions when compared to the non-taxi driver group (see Figure 7.1 on p. C2). These regions were the left and right hippocampi. No other brain regions differed. Further analysis focusing on the hippocampal region revealed that there was an increased volume of grey matter in the *posterior* part of both the left and right hippocampus of taxi drivers compared to the control group. This was in contrast to the *anterior* part of both left and right hippocampi, whose grey matter volume was decreased in taxi drivers.

The authors conducted a further set of analyses and correlated the amount of time spent by each of the 16 participants working as a taxi driver (i.e., their working experience) with the volume of grey matter. They found that the length of time spent as a taxi driver correlated positively with volume of grey matter in the posterior hippocampus (Figure 7.1). That is, the more experienced the taxi driver, the greater the volume of grey matter in the posterior hippocampus. At the same time the authors also found a concomitant experience-related decrease in the volume of grey matter in the anterior hippocampus (Figure 7.2).

This study is important for a number of reasons. In the broadest terms, it provides a very clear demonstration that particular regions of the brain are 'devoted' to certain cognitive tasks, in this case spatial memory for navigation. The authors even go so far as to suggest that a mental map of London may be stored in the posterior part of the hippocampus of these taxi drivers. This in itself may not be particularly new or

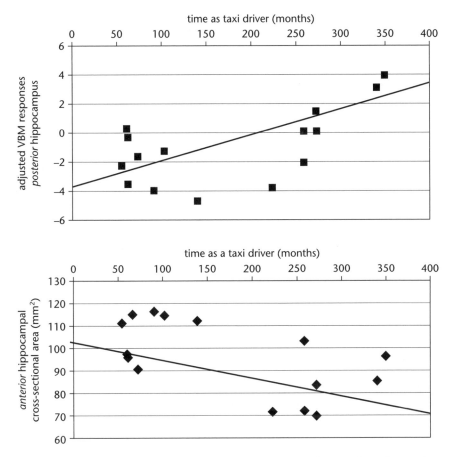

Figure 7.2 Correlation of volume change with time as a taxi driver. The volume of grey matter in the right hippocampus was found to correlate significantly with the amount of time spent learning to be and practising as a licensed London taxi driver, positively in the right posterior hippocampus (top) and negatively in the anterior hippocampus (bottom).

Source: Reprinted with permission from the National Academy of Science: *PNAS* (Maguire et al., 2000), © (2000).

remarkable; many other studies have previously identified regions of cortex specifically associated with distinct mental operations such as language comprehension, face perception, motor control and vigilance (to name a few). But the beauty of this study is that it rests on a group of normal individuals whose daily profession has afforded them a unique proficiency in one particular cognitive domain – spatial memory. As such, the study is free from much of the artifice that can cast a shadow over the validity of many laboratory-based experiments and tests; this group of London taxi drivers represent a refreshing antidote to the typical population of undergraduate students learning word lists or stimulus pairs who usually populate such studies in the literature. In effect, this study brings the neural correlates of mental capacities into a real-world context in a way that is rarely seen in the literature.

A second important implication of the findings is the suggestion that the structure of the brain is malleable and subject to use-dependent plastic change; this is revealed most dramatically in the correlations between the taxi drivers' length of time in the job and hippocampal volume change. Other work on neural plasticity has shown that with experience comes a rearrangement of the brain's circuitry and physical connectivity (see Chapter 2). While many of these studies demonstrate this sort of plasticity in primary motor or sensory cortices, the taxi driver study hints strongly that the same type of structural or volumetric change may occur in regions of the brain devoted to *higher-order functioning* (e.g. spatial memory in this case). This carries very important implications for a number of areas. In terms of rehabilitation, this finding provides great encouragement for the possibility of recovery from brain injury impacting on higher-order cognitive capacities. Furthermore, brain change as a result of prolonged experience or learning may provide an avenue by which the elderly can maintain their neural, and in parallel, cognitive health into later life. Regimes of memory or attention training and mental exercise have been shown to alter brain chemistry in specific structures, thereby leading to increases in cell viability and integrity. Such interventions may represent an effective approach to reducing the risk of dementia and other age-related cognitive decline. Finally, the results suggest an insight into the types of structural change that take place in the brain as one progresses from novice to expert status in any field of activity.

Another thought-provoking issue that arises from this study is the fact that changes in one part of the brain have implications for other parts of the brain. As we can see from the taxi drivers' data, although there is an increase in the posterior region of their hippocampus, simultaneously there is a decrease in grey matter volume in the anterior region. So, in effect, the flipside to the growth in the posterior hippocampal area that seems to be driven by repeated use and activity is the expansion of this region into the anatomical space occupied by its anterior counterpart. Again, such coopting of adjacent areas when plastic change causes a cortical region to expand has been observed elsewhere in the plasticity literature for both motor (e.g. Plautz et al., 2000) and sensory cortical areas (Polley et al., 2006), or following the amputation of a limb, in which neighbouring cortical areas encroach on the now unused sensory or motor regions (see Chen et al., 2002). However, the demonstration of this apparent trade-off with regard to a higher-order cognitive process poses the troublesome question – does this expansion of posterior hippocampus at the apparent expense of the anterior portion of the same structure lead to an associated deficit in the cognitive activities underpinned by anterior hippocampus? And if so, are these impairments manifested behaviourally?

It is because of the combination of several features that this study can be considered innovative and important: the clarity of hypothesis and design; the use of an ethologically valid sample of everyday people; the rigour of analysis in using two independent indices of brain volume change; the compelling simplicity of the results; the many implications raised by the findings. For these main reasons, we would view Maguire et al. (2000) as a pioneering study in the cognitive neuroscience of memory.

Author commentary by Eleanor A. Maguire

I remember clearly walking into Chris Frith's office over 10 years ago, and him shaking his head in understandable disbelief. . . . 'It'll never work; they won't agree to be scanned'. With blissful naivety I persevered with the attempt to understand the neural basis of navigation in humans, and in particular the role of the hippocampus. The problem at the time was this; it was difficult to find people with the same level of experience of one particular environment to be subjects in functional neuroimaging experiments. Thus, in order to have experimental control, learning of new environments (by watching videos or using virtual reality; Maguire et al., 1996, 1998) was employed instead. However, most of our everyday activities take place in familiar environments, learned over many years that we need to navigate constantly. It was imperative, therefore, to find a way to assess this. I had seen on television a programme about licensed London taxi drivers, their training (colloquially known as acquiring 'The Knowledge'), the area whose layout they needed to learn – 25,000 London streets including thousands of places of interest, and the stringent examinations set by the Public Carriage Office (PCO) that must be passed in order to obtain an operating licence. Here was what I had been looking for, a group of people with a verified level of knowledge of the same environment acquired over a number of years; but would they be scanned? Yes – then, and to this day, the licensed taxi drivers of London and the PCO have enabled what could be regarded as a unique research opportunity.

The initial interest in 1997 was to use functional imaging to examine brain areas activated while taxi drivers mentally navigated along routes in London (Maguire et al., 1997). Around this time, reading a review by Lee et al. (1998), I was reminded that spatial memory in non-humans (e.g. food-catching birds and mammals) was also associated with structural brain differences, and increased hippocampal volume with increased demands on spatial memory. Researchers were also starting to publish exciting work showing clear evidence for neurogenesis in the hippocampus in non-humans and (in post-mortem tissue) in humans (Kempermann et al., 1997, 1998; Eriksson et al., 1998; Gould et al., 1999). This offered a possible mechanism for the structural changes in animals.

It was at this point that I wondered if humans who have placed a great demand on their spatial memory might also show structural brain changes. It was relatively easy to gather structural MRI scans on willing taxi drivers, but how to measure hippocampal volume was more challenging. Up until then this was typically accomplished by region of interest (ROI) methods. A trained observer would manually trace around the hippocampus on an MRI scan, scan slice by slice, and then calculate the volume of the structure (Van Paesschen et al., 1997). However, this technique is open to observer bias, is extremely time-consuming, restricted to specific regions and not suitable to interrogate the whole brain. Thus, the final ingredient that enabled the Maguire et al. (2000) study was the timely development of a new method for analysing structural MRI brain scans. Voxel-based morphometry (VBM) (Wright et al., 1995; May et al., 1999) was entirely automated and permitted examination of the whole brain. Since its development it had been mostly used to study grey and white matter volume differences in clinical populations, but I thought it would be interesting to use with taxi drivers. The question was would VBM be sufficiently sensitive to detect subtle differences in the context of healthy brains?

I have to be honest and say I did not expect to see any grey matter volume differences between taxi driver brains and those of control subjects. So I was shocked when it was clearly evident that the posterior hippocampi had a greater grey matter volume in taxi drivers, the anterior hippocampi intriguingly had less volume, and these volumes correlated with time spent taxi driving (see Figures 7.1 and 7.2). So sceptical was I that I asked David Gadian at the Institute of Child Health at University College London (UCL) to take the scans and independently and blindly apply the traditional ROI method to see if the results concurred, and they did. It seemed that learning, storing and using a complex spatial representation of a large city was associated with hippocampal grey matter differences in taxi drivers. Furthermore, the correlation between hippocampal grey matter volume and time spent taxi driving suggested these changes were *acquired*.

The taxi driver study had important implications generally, as well as personally for my own work. In general, the findings, although cross-sectional, added new fuel to the nature versus nurture debate. An enduring question in memory research is just how plastic is the brain's memory system? Can we drive it and invariably achieve improved performance, or are there limits, and if so, what are the influencing factors? Addressing these questions is important as the answers will have universal relevance by informing what each of us can hope to achieve, may have important implications for education and, crucially, for patients with memory impairments. If we are to approach rehabilitation in a systematic and efficacious way, then it is vital to know if the memory system has the propensity for plasticity in adulthood, the limiting factors on such plasticity, and the time-scales of any plastic change. There had been previous reports of the volume of some brain areas in humans being different in groups with special skills; for example planum temporale in musicians (Schlaug et al., 1995). However in cases such as these (and bilingualism – Mechelli et al., 2004) the skills were usually acquired in childhood, thus conflating brain development and skill acquisition. The taxi drivers, by contrast, only started their intensive training and navigation in adulthood, and their data seem to suggest that environmentally stimulated plasticity in the adult human brain can occur. The study also provided some intriguing insights into possible mechanisms of plasticity, in that a brain region did not just get bigger; it did so at the cost of grey matter volume elsewhere, implying that plasticity may be a story of loss as well as gain. This study, by testing VBM with an independent method and showing that it could be used to detect subtle volume differences in healthy brains, also helped to popularize VBM, and since then there has been an explosion of VBM studies looking at a variety of cognitive and psychological factors, as well as its ongoing use in clinical populations.

In terms of my own research, the taxi driver study provided key evidence in my quest to understand the role of the human hippocampus, and sparked a set of follow-up cross-sectional studies (Maguire et al., 2003a, b; Maguire et al., 2006; Woollett and Maguire, 2009). As well as twice replicating the original finding, we also established that while taxi drivers excelled on London-based knowledge tests, they were significantly worse on anterograde memory tests involving associative processing (Maguire et al., 2006; Woollett and Maguire, 2009). These findings offer insights into the likely functions of the anterior hippocampi, where the volume is less in taxi drivers. Moreover, they are suggestive of limits in the capacity for expression of hippocampal plasticity such that spatial expertise is offset by a cost to certain kinds of new memories. Interestingly, we found no such effects on neuropsychological performance or grey matter volume when we tested experts who had acquired large amounts of non-spatial knowledge (Woollett et al., 2008), thus suggesting a special role for the hippocampus in representing space.

Correlations between time taxi driving and hippocampal grey matter in the cross-sectional studies suggest that navigation experience drives the changes observed. In order to directly examine this we are currently engaged in a longitudinal study whereby trainee London taxi drivers are being tracked from when they start their course of learning ('The Knowledge', which takes 2–4 years) until qualification. The final results will allow us to examine if the hippocampus shows genuine *within-subjects* plasticity in response to navigation experience. Even then the taxi driver story will not be complete. It may be possible to assess whether the propensity for plasticity is genetically influenced (Egan et al., 2003; Hariri et al., 2003), adding further important evidence into the nature/nurture debate. Recent developments in magnetic resonance (MR) spectroscopy may mean that we can penetrate grey matter beyond the level of VBM, and image neurogenesis in vivo in the human brain (Manganas et al., 2007).

Thus, from a simple initial idea, it has proved fruitful to use the London taxi driver model as a means from which to extract general principles about the boundaries within which human memory operates. But the effects of the study were not just scientific. When the paper was first published it made the front page of every major newspaper in the UK and many around the world. I was inundated with requests for television, radio and magazine interviews. Not a day goes by even now when there isn't a telephone call or email from the media wanting to talk about 'the taxi driver work', and most recently the study has found its way onto the UK school curriculum and is now on the A-level psychology syllabus. Clearly, it struck a chord in the public mind. There seems to be an enduring fascination with memory, but much of neuroscience is difficult to engage with. The appeal, therefore, of the Maguire et al. (2000) study may be the way in which it managed to genuinely combine scientific merit with general accessibility, something that happens perhaps all too rarely.

Peer commentary by Shane M. O'Mara

Significance

During October 2008, Maguire et al. (2000) had 464 citations on Google Scholar and 299 on the Web of Science. This is a remarkable rate of citation for what at first glance is a somewhat esoteric topic – a study of the brains of London's taxi drivers. Why would studying the brains of taxi drivers be at all interesting, beyond the brains of lawyers or computer scientists or mechanics or even those of neuroscientists? The rate at which this paper is cited in the scientific literature suggests that there is already a general judgement that this is a significant and important piece of work. There are many criteria by which the importance of a paper can be assessed. The standard international criteria revolve around metrics such as citations of the paper and, as we have seen, these are amply fulfilled. There are other more informal and less quantitative criteria, however, applied by the working researcher to new findings in the literature. One mark of the importance of a paper is its obviousness – and by obviousness I mean the obviousness created only by the gift of hindsight. A breakthrough paper should come with the feeling after you have read it that 'I should have done this study – it was obvious (or the findings/data were obvious) . . .' (but of course the study was not obvious beforehand, nor were the findings/data!).

Another important mark is that of bifurcation – what we thought before, and what we think now, has changed and cannot be changed back – in fact it becomes hard to remember what it was you thought before! Another mark is fruitfulness – how many new ideas or ways of thinking about fundamental mechanisms does it lead to or how many doors to new experiments does it open? The creative use of a naturalistic experimental sample of convenience, available in some numbers because of peculiar circumstance, is another particular mark of the importance of this paper. By any or all of these criteria, Maguire et al. (2000) is a very significant paper indeed. Here, I sketch some of the reasons why this paper is a significant, indeed, landmark paper in cognitive neuroscience.

Implications

Hebb (1949) famously argued that activity-dependent change is at the heart of memory formation in the brain. Hebb's two-part formulation states, first, that '. . . a reverberatory trace might cooperate with structural change, and carry the memory until the growth change is made . . .' and, second, that 'when an axon of cell A is near enough to excite a cell B and repeatedly or persistently takes part in firing it, some growth process or metabolic change takes place in one or both cells so that A's efficiency as one of the cells firing B is increased'. Maguire et al. (2000) provide a key vindication of Hebb's hypothesis that some growth process underlies activity-dependent memory formation in the *adult* brain. Thus, functional (cognitive) activity, when sustained for a sufficiently long period, is converted into a structural change in the brain, allowing memories to be more-or-less indefinitely retained by the brain. What Maguire et al. demonstrate is that the adult brain is plastic, and can be structurally reorganized as the result of sustained experience (i.e. plasticity is activity-dependent).

The result here is in one sense obvious – somebody should have conducted a study of this type with such a specialized population before, but crucially no one did. And the results – they were obvious too (but only in retrospect). The history of neuroscience from Cajal up to the 1970s provides us with few enough studies that give us the locus of the engram (the specific location of memory-related changes in the brain). Here, we have a specific and experience- rather than pathology-, drug- or developmental-related change that results in the structural expansion of the brain. The picture that develops is the brain as muscle – with cognitive effort resulting in expansion of a key brain area concerned with supporting a particular type of memory.

Limitations

Every study has its limitations, and there are many associated with Maguire et al., 2000 – but as these were not part of the research focus, then these limitations might be better thought of as the next study to do. Maguire et al. throw no light on the well-known male–female differences in spatial cognition (Kimura, 1999), for example, perhaps because of the dearth of female taxi drivers. The first obvious limitation of Maguire et al. is that it is not a functional brain imaging study – it does not address how changes in functional inputs lead to widespread structural reorganization in a particular (but predicted) brain region. This was not the particular intent of the study, however, so this is not an entirely reasonable criticism. But the question remains – do the structural changes lead to functional advantages? The answer appears to be yes – taxi drivers appear to have exceptional memories for street names, for example, compared to normal controls (Kalakoski and Saariluoma, 2001). This exceptional memory presumably has a structural basis rooted in the changes observed by Maguire et al.; their study is silent as to the nature of the underlying physiological changes that eventuate in these substantial regional structural changes. Further brain imaging studies focused on regional metabolic differences or on brain connectivity might expose the underlying mechanisms supporting this form of activity-dependent change, as might studies combining functional genomics with brain imaging (Egan et al., 2003). The neural locus of memory and how it changes through time is not addressed by this study either: Rosenbaum et al. (2005) found that a former-Toronto-based taxi driver with extensive atrophy of the hippocampus, resulting from Alzheimer's disease, performed at the level of controls (including an encephalitis patient) on remote memory tests of spatial location and mental navigation between well-known Toronto landmarks (which he had not visited for at least a decade, after his retirement). Thus, perhaps some degree of protection or resilience against the loss of certain classes of previously learned items in memory is conferred by repetitive exposure to, and practice of navigating through, a complex urban environment against subsequent insult caused by Alzheimer's disease.

A curious and less-remarked upon result of Maguire et al. (2000) revolves around the differential change seen between anterior and posterior hippocampi of taxi drivers versus non-taxi drivers. It appears that grey matter in the right posterior hippocampus correlated significantly with time spent as a taxi driver (Fig 7.2, top), but negatively in the anterior hippocampus (Fig 7.2, bottom). Thus, the positive conclusion of Maguire et al. ('. . . local plasticity in the structure of the healthy adult human brain as a function of increasing exposure to an environmental stimulus' p. 4402) is well-founded. What explains the opposite result – that there is a decrease in grey matter volume in anterior hippocampus that follows the length of time spent as a taxi driver? Sadly, there are too many alternative explanations to directly interpret this result. The continuing and unrelieved stress of being a driver in a very busy city might be at fault; for example, the hippocampus is particularly vulnerable to the effects of stress hormones (Lupien et al., 1998). Another possibility is that there is a ceiling effect present, given by the brain itself – that increases in volume in one part of a structure might somehow be balanced by a decrease in volume in another, perhaps caused by the persistent shunt of metabolic resources along the longitudinal axis of the hippocampus. This difference remains unexplained, and will be a fruitful source of further investigation in the future.

Open questions

Maguire et al. 2002 conclude with the following statement: 'It remains to be seen whether similar environment-related plasticity is possible in other regions of the human brain outside of the hippocampus'. I have alluded to the well-known differences in spatial cognition between males and females, with the advantage accruing to males. What is the origin of this difference? Is it a genetic given, like eye colour, or is it something else, such as motivation? If this capacity is plastic, then task-practice should reduce or eliminate these male–female differences. Feng et al. (2007) have conducted a remarkable experiment suggesting that it is the latter. They found that a training regime, playing an action video game for 10 hours, reduced dramatically the differences observed between males and females in spatial cognition, assessed by tasks focused on mental rotation, compared to subjects who played non-action video games. This study implies that if a sufficiently large group of female London taxi drivers were available to Maguire that there would be no structural differences between their posterior hippocampi; further, there should be no differences in spatial cognition either. Time on task is probably the key variable here, accounting for a substantial fraction of the variance, rather than gender. A fascinating study would be to combine this innovative cognitive psychology experiment with structural and functional brain imaging – to discover the locus of the change within the brain, and also to measure how the change itself occurs and evolves over time.

Conclusions

Maguire et al. 2000 have provided a bookend to the now outdated view that the adult human brain has limited or no capacity for structural plasticity. They show that by creatively thinking and focusing on a special naturalistically available sample, difficult questions can be answered, and answered in a way that suggests many new questions that can be very profitably explored. There may be other such populations available (middle-aged or elderly adopters of new technologies or musical instruments, for example) to be profitably investigated, especially if other convergent methodologies are adopted, such as functional brain imaging, genomics or experimental cognitive psychology.

References

Chen, R., Cohen, L.G. and Hallett, M. (2002) Nervous system reorganization following injury, *Neuroscience*, 111(4): 761–73.

Corkin, S. (2002) What's new with the amnesic patient H.M.? *Nature Reviews Neuroscience*, 3(2): 153–60.

Egan, M.F., Kojima, M., Callicott, J.H. et al. (2003) The BDNF val66met polymorphism affects activity-dependent secretion of BDNF and human memory and hippocampal function, *Cell*, 112: 257–69.

Eriksson, P.S., Perfilieva, E., Bjork-Eriksson, T. et al. (1998) Neurogenesis in the adult human hippocampus, *Nature Medicine*, 4: 1313–17.

Feng, J., Spence, I. and Pratt, J. (2007) Playing an action video game reduces gender differences in spatial cognition, *Psychological Science*, 18: 850–5.

Gould, E., Beylin, A., Tanapat, P., Reeves, A. and Shors, T. (1999) Learning enhances adult neurogenesis in the hippocampal formation, *Nature Neuroscience*, 2: 260–5.

Hariri, A.R., Goldberg, T., Mattay, V.S. et al. (2003) Brain-derived neurotrophic factor val66met polymorphism affects human memory-related hippocampal activity and predicts memory performance, *Journal of Neuroscience*, 23: 6690–4.

Hebb, D.O. (1949) *The Organization of Behaviour*. New York: Wiley.

Kalakoski, V. and Saariluoma, P. (2001) Taxi drivers' exceptional memory of street names, *Memory & Cognition*, 29: 634–8.

Kempermann, G., Kuhn, H.G. and Gage, F.H. (1997) More hippocampal neurons in adult mice living in an enriched environment, *Nature*, 386: 493–5.

Kempermann, G., Kuhn, H.G. and Gage, F.H. (1998) Experience-induced neurogenesis in the senescent dentate gyrus, *Journal of Neuroscience*, 18: 3206–12.

Kimura, D. (1999) *Sex and Cognition*. Cambridge, MA: MIT Press.

Lee, D.W., Miyasato, L.E. and Clayton, N.S. (1998) Neurobiological bases of spatial learning in the natural environment: neurogenesis and growth in the avian and mammalian hippocampus, *NeuroReport*, 9: R15–R27.

Lupien, S.J., de Leon, M., de Santi, S. et al. (1998) Cortisol levels during human aging predict hippocampal atrophy and memory deficits, *Nature Neuroscience*, 1: 69–73.

Maguire, E.A., Frackowiak, R.S.J. and Frith, C.D. (1996) Learning to find your way – a role for the human hippocampal region, *Proceedings of the Royal Society of London*, Series B, 263: 1745–50.

Maguire, E.A., Frackowiak, R.S.J. and Frith, C.D. (1997) Recalling routes around London: activation of the right hippocampus in taxi drivers, *Journal of Neuroscience*, 17: 7103–10.

Maguire, E.A., Burgess, N., Donnett, J.G. et al. (1998) Knowing where and getting there: a human navigation network, *Science*, 280: 921–4.

Maguire, E.A., Gadian, D.G., Johnsrude, I.S. et al. (2000) Navigation-related structural change in the hippocampi of taxi drivers, *Proceedings of the National Academy of Sciences, USA*, 97: 4398–403.

Maguire, E.A., Spiers, H.J., Good, C.D. et al. (2003a) Navigation expertise and the human hippocampus: a structural brain imaging analysis, *Hippocampus*, 13: 208–17.

Maguire, E.A., Valentine, E.R., Wilding, J.M. and Kapur, N. (2003b) Routes to remembering: the brains behind superior memory, *Nature Neuroscience*, 6: 90–5.

Maguire, E.A., Woollett, K. and Spiers, H.J. (2006) London taxi drivers and bus drivers: a structural MRI and neuropsychological analysis, *Hippocampus*, 16: 1091–101.

Manganas, L.N., Zhang, X., Li, Y. et al. (2007) Magnetic resonance spectroscopy identifies neural progenitor cells in the live human brain, *Science*, 318: 980–5.

May, A., Ashburner, J., Büchel, C. et al. (1999) Correlation between structural and functional changes in brain in an idiopathic headache syndrome, *Nature Medicine*, 5: 836–8.

Mechelli, A., Crinion, J.T., Noppeney, U. et al. (2004) Neurolinguistics: structural plasticity in the bilingual brain, *Nature*, 431: 757.

O'Keefe, J. and Dostrovsky, J. (1971) The hippocampus as a spatial map: preliminary evidence from unit activity in the freely-moving rat, *Brain Research*, 34(1): 171–5.

Plautz, E.J., Milliken, G.W. and Nudo, R.J. (2000) Effects of repetitive motor training on movement representations in adult squirrel monkeys: role of use versus learning, *Neurobiology of Learning and Memory*, 74(1): 27–55.

Polley, D.B., Steinberg, E.E. and Merzenich, M.M. (2006) Perceptual learning directs auditory cortical map reorganization through top-down influences, *Journal of Neuroscience*, 26(18): 4970–82.

Rosenbaum, R.S., Gao, F., Richards, B., Black, S.E. and Moscovitch, M. (2005) 'Where to?' remote memory for spatial relations and landmark identity in former taxi drivers with Alzheimer's disease and encephalitis, *Journal of Cognitive Neuroscience*, 17(3): 446–62.

Schlaug, G., Jancke, L., Huang, Y. and Steinmetz, H. (1995) In vivo evidence of structural brain asymmetry in musicians, *Science*, 267: 699–701.

Scoville, W.B. and Milner, B. (1957) Loss of recent memory after bilateral hippocampal lesions, *Journal of Neurology, Neurosurgery and Psychiatry*, 20(1): 11–21.

Smulders, T.V., Sasson, A.D. and DeVoogd, T.J. (1995) Seasonal variation in hippocampal volume in a food-storing bird, the black-capped chickadee, *Journal of Neurobiology*, 27(1): 15–25.

Van Paesschen, W., Connolly, A., King, M.D., Jackson, G.D. and Duncan, J.S. (1997) The spectrum of hippocampal sclerosis: a quantitative magnetic resonance imaging study, *Annals of Neurology*, 41: 41–51.

Woollett, K., Glensman, J. and Maguire, E.A. (2008) Non-spatial expertise and hippocampal gray matter volume in humans, *Hippocampus*, 18(10): 981–4.

Woollett, K. and Maguire, E.A. (2009) Navigational expertise may compromise anterograde associative memory, *Neuropsychologia*, 47(4): 1088–95.

Wright, I.C., McGuire, P.K., Poline, J.-B. et al. (1995) A voxel-based method for the statistical analysis of gray and white matter density applied to schizophrenia, *Neuroimage*, 2: 244–52.

8   Crossed wires in the brain: multisensory integration in synaesthesia

Discussion of:

Esterman, M., Verstynen, T., Ivry, R.B. and Robertson, L.C. (2006)

Coming unbound: disrupting automatic integration of synesthetic color and graphemes by TMS of the right parietal lobe, *Journal of Cognitive Neuroscience*, 18(9): 1570–6

Reprinted with permission from MIT Press © 2006

Foreword, background and description by Richard A.P. Roche and Seán Commins
Author's commentary by Lynn Robertson
Peer commentary by John Foxe

Foreword

Synaesthesia is a relatively rare condition in which a person's sensory systems appear to effectively *cross over* in an unusual way; specifically, a particular experience in one sensory modality will automatically elicit a sensation in a different sense modality. Some forms of synaesthesia involve the experience of a specific taste when a person hears a certain sound, or the feeling of a certain shape when a word or letter is presented. More common among synaesthetes is a cross-over between vision and hearing, resulting in colours being evoked for certain numbers, letters or words (termed 'colour-grapheme synaesthesia'). The neural origins of synaesthesia may be related to some cross-wiring in the implicated sensory systems, though the precise underpinnings are not yet well understood. In this chapter, we describe an experiment that investigates the role of the posterior parietal cortex in colour-grapheme synaesthesia using repetitive-pulse transcranial magnetic stimulation (rTMS), a methodological approach that can temporarily inhibit the functioning of (or effectively create a temporary lesion in) a brain area while participants perform a task. The use of such 'virtual lesion' technology in this study allows the potential involvement of the posterior parietal cortex in synaesthetic binding to be examined, making this a pioneering study in the cognitive neuroscience of synaesthesia.

Introduction

At any moment in time, our brains are carrying out many complex translations. In our visual system, the jumble of light or dark blobs and the scattered patches of colour that arrive at our eyes are converted into objects and surfaces, edges and boundaries by an array of sophisticated processes. Higher up in this system, the two-dimensional image that we see is translated into a three-dimensional representation of the world, complete with depth perception and an understanding of which objects are in front of, or are behind, others. Our auditory system converts the vibrations of our ear-drums into sounds of different pitch, tone and frequency, while other processes within this system translate these sounds into meaningful words or phrases that can trigger stored representations of objects, people or events in our memory. Many of these processes occur almost instantaneously or automatically, and often it is only when they fail that we even notice their presence at all, as in the case of impaired perception of colour, or *cerebral achromatopsia*.

Reading, in particular, is a capacity that requires many such translations; first, to identify each letter correctly and then to attribute the associated sound to that particular letter. By adulthood, the association of a particular sound with each letter of the alphabet has become, for most of us, relatively instantaneous – the presentation of the letter 'R' will, for example, elicit the appropriate 'r-sound' in a virtually automatic manner. While seemingly effortless and not particularly unusual, this ability that allows a visual object (a letter) to evoke a particular sound (the associated phoneme) is actually an example of cross-modal processing – a sensation in the visual domain evokes an experience not physically present in the auditory. In synaesthetes, similar forms of sensory transfer occur automatically across some unexpected combinations of sensory domains – sounds can evoke colours, tastes can evoke tactile sensations and visual stimuli can elicit smells. In fact, in synaesthesia, cross-modal transfer can take place for any pair of sense modalities, although the most common form appears to be coloured hearing.

Research into synaesthesia goes back as far as Sir Francis Galton (1822–1911), a first cousin to Charles Darwin and an early pioneer of psychology. During his attempts in the 1880s to conduct rigorous psychometric profiling of the population, he discovered many people for whom letters or words evoked the sensation of a particular colour; often these were days of the week or months of the year, although individual letters or numbers were also found to elicit colour sensations. Galton also noted that some people represented numbers in unusual spatial arrangements, a phenomenon he referred to as 'number forms'. For some, this consisted of the numbers being arranged in a spiral formation around the body; for others, they were represented by abstract shapes. Subsequent research termed the condition 'synaesthesia', and it was found that such experiences are not uncommon in the population, with a prevalence 1 in 20 people according to some estimates.[1] While the within-modality colour-grapheme synaesthesia (i.e. coloured letters, numbers, days or months) appears to be the most frequently observed type, rarer forms such as vision-evoking tastes or tactile sensations have also been closely studied. Different theories of synaesthesia have been proposed; some suggest that neural cross-wiring in sensory cortices may be responsible for coloured hearing or tasting shapes, while others claim that more abstract types of synaesthesia, such as personalities for letters or shapes for numbers, may be due to the formation of unusually strong associations during critical periods of childhood development.

Theoretical viewpoints notwithstanding, genetic studies have confirmed that synaes-thesia seems to run in families and may have a strong genetic basis (e.g. Barnett et al., 2008a), while imaging studies of synaesthetes have demonstrated activations of colour-associated regions of visual cortex (area V4) during elicited synaesthetic visual sensations as a result of non-visual stimulus presentation (e.g. Sperling et al., 2006; Hubbard et al., 2005). These lines of research confirm that synaesthesia is a genuine sensory experience on the part of the synaesthetes and possibly a heritable condition. Some have even gone so far as to suggest that the ability to carry out synaesthetic-like translations is what allowed us to develop a written language in our evolutionary past, where specific visual symbols became capable of evoking the particular sound associ-ated with that symbol. As such, the capacity for synaesthetic experience is something that we all share.

In the study described in this chapter, Esterman and colleagues carried out an experi-ment with two colour-grapheme synaesthetes, each of whom had a distinct set of colours associated with each letter of the alphabet. Taking into account the coloured alphabet of each participant, the experimenters presented letters of the alphabet on screen in either a colour that matched that of their synaesthetic experience (congru-ent), or in a different colour to that automatically elicited by that letter (incongruent). All participants had to do was press a button to indicate the actual colour in which the letter was presented. Often, synaesthetes performing this type of task show faster responses when the presented colour is congruent to their synaesthetic experience of the letter, while slower responses are frequently seen for incongruent trials as they try to inhibit the evoked colour and concentrate on the colour actually present. These response times are usually compared to control stimuli that do not evoke synaesthetic responses (such as #, % and &) presented in different colours.

Using this paradigm, Esterman and colleagues wanted to investigate the possible role of a part of posterior parietal cortex in synaesthetic binding. It had already been demonstrated that the experience of synaesthetically evoked colours results in activa-tion of visual areas associated with colour perception (see above), but other studies had reported activations in poster parietal areas during such experiences. These areas were suspected of involvement in the binding of sensory stimulations such as colour and shape; this had been shown previously in synaesthetes and non-synaesthetes alike as they combined colour and shape information (Donner et al., 2002). Other studies also suggested a role for the posterior parietal cortex (PPC) in perceptual binding of this sort, both in normals and synaesthetes. To investigate whether the PPC is function-ally significant in such colour-shape binding, Esterman and colleagues employed a methodological technique that can reveal whether an area of the brain is necessary for the execution of a cognitive operation, unlike brain imaging, which merely shows cortical regions that are active during a task (and is therefore correlational). This advantageous type of information, termed 'functional resolution' by its exponents, is provided by the technique of transcranial magnetic stimulation (TMS).

TMS involves the application of large and quickly changing magnetic fields in the vicinity of the cerebral cortex. The rapid reversal of polarity of this large magnetic field has the effect of inducing cell firing in any cortical tissue near the point of focus of the magnetic field. We have already seen how TMS can be used to map portions of motor or sensory cortex associated with particular body parts (see Chapter 2), but an additional application of TMS is its use as a 'virtual lesion' technique. Induced cell firing due to TMS near the scalp can effectively 'knock out' the involvement of a cortical region within a processing loop, effectively causing a temporary and transient (hence 'virtual') brain lesion. In this way, neuroscientists can investigate whether a particular brain area is *necessary for* (rather than associated with) the execution of a cognitive task. In a typical TMS study, the involvement of a region in a task will be indicated by slower reaction times than normal when the TMS pulses are applied, as the effect of the repetitive pulses is to temporarily block processing in that cortical circuit (for a detailed description of TMS, its principles and uses, see Walsh and Pascual-Leone, 2003). In the present study, the authors hypothesized that rTMS applied to the PPC would interfere with the normal synaesthetic binding process, thereby abolishing the slowed response times usually seen for incongruent trials.

Background and description of the study

Two participants with colour–grapheme synaesthesia took part in this study. In colour–grapheme synaesthesia, particular graphemes are perceived in specific colours. For example, the letter 'A' is always seen in a particular shade of red, while the letter 'B' is perceived as blue. Both participants were female and right-handed with CP being 27 years old at the time of the study and EF being 22. Both participants reported as having specific alphanumeric–colour associations that showed long-term stability. In the case of EF, for example, the letter 'A' is perceived as red, while 'B' is seen as a shade of green (see Figure 8.1 on p. C3 for the full synaesthetic alphabet for EF).

Before testing, each participant was requested to sit at approximately 30cm in front of a computer screen. An alphanumeric symbol was then presented on the screen and each participant was required to adjust the screen colour so that the RGB screen value matched that of the current stimulus according to their synaesthetic alphabet. For example, if the number '6' appeared on the screen, EF readjusted the colour of the screen so that it matched the pink colour that she perceived.

The authors wished to determine whether short-term inhibition of the parietal cortex would reduce the participant's synaesthetic tendencies. The parietal cortex was chosen as this region is known to contribute to the binding of colour and shape in synaesthesia. In order to evoke this transient inhibition in the parietal cortex, rTMS was used. Each participant was subjected to either rTMS or sham rTMS (in which the TMS coil was oriented away from the scalp so no pulses were directed towards the underlying brain tissue but the sound and tactile sensation were the same). The participants did not know whether they were receiving sham or real stimulation. Each rTMS period consisted of 480 consecutive pulses that were delivered at a rate of 1 Hz (eight minutes in total). Both left and right parietal cortices were targeted. Stimulation was delivered to the angular gyrus at the junction of the posterior intraparietal sulcus and transverse occipital sulcus (IPS and TOS, respectively) of the parietal cortex bilaterally, using each participant's individual MRI scan as the basis for localization (see Figure 8.2 on p. C3), for targeted IPS/TOS site in the MRI scan for EF). Repetitive TMS was also applied over the primary visual cortex (V1) as a control region and to test for the effects of generalized tissue stimulation on responses in the colour-naming task.

Following TMS, each participant was then given a colour-naming task. Here, each participant was presented with a series of letters that was either in a colour that was congruent or incongruent to their own synaesthetic photism. For example, on congruent trials, participant EF was presented with the letters J, M and O in green, purple and white, respectively. On the incongruent trials these same letters were presented in alternative colours. A third series of neutral stimuli in different colours was also presented (these symbols did not provoke a synaesthetic response (see Figure 8.3 on p. C4 for examples of the three trial types given to participant EF). All trials were presented randomly to each participant, who were required to name the colour of the grapheme as quickly as possible. Two blocks of trials were given; an early block and a late block. The early block was given 1–5 minutes post-stimulation and the late block was given 6–10 minutes post-stimulation. It was expected that the stimulation effect would have worn off by the late block.

It would be expected under 'normal' (synaesthetic) circumstances that the participants' reaction times would be significantly slower on incongruent compared to both congruent and neutral trials, as they would try to suppress their synaesthetic photism. However, it was hypothesized that rTMS applied to the parietal lobe would attenuate this effect by facilitating the binding of the presented colour grapheme.

Results from both EF and CP suggest that, with sham rTMS, reaction times were slower on the incongruent trials compared to the other two trial types, as was expected. This was true independent of the location of stimulation and timing of testing (early or late). For example, in the case of CP, following sham stimulation of the right parietal lobe, reaction times (for the early block) on the incongruent trials were slower (647 +/– 186 ms) compared to both the congruent (574 +/– 158 ms) and neutral trials (615 +/– 161 ms). Similarly for EF, following sham stimulation of the left parietal lobe, reaction times (for the late block) on the incongruent trials were slower (529 +/– 119 ms) than both congruent (462 +/– 94 ms) and neutral trials (496 +/– 90 ms). However, with rTMS (non-sham) over the right parietal lobe reaction times were not significantly different on the incongruent trials when compared to both congruent and neutral trial types. This effect was observed irrespective of the timing of testing: following rTMS of EF's right parietal lobe, early block reaction times on the incongruent trials were no different (497 +/– 96 ms) to congruent (423 +/– 58 ms) or neutral trials (481 +/– 88 ms). A similar pattern was observed for CP. Interestingly, this attenuation of the synaesthetic photism interference effect was not observed when stimulation was applied to the left parietal lobe; for EF following stimulation of the left parietal lobe, early block reaction times for incongruent trials were longer (530 +/– 141 ms) compared to both congruent (449 +/– 93 ms) and neutral trials (469 +/– 84 ms). As would be expected, the attenuation effect was not observed following the control V1 stimulation.

These results can be summarized by graphing the interference effect for both participants; Figure 8.4 demonstrates that, for both EF and CP, stimulation over the right parietal lobe attenuates (as indicated by negative-going grey bars) the interference effect that is normally observed. Stimulation of both the left parietal lobe and V1 does not show such attenuation.

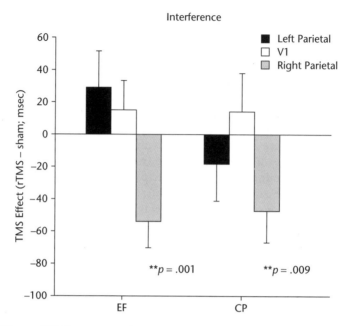

Figure 8.4 Effects of TMS on synaesthetic interference. Bar chart demonstrates the effects of rTMS on synaesthetic interference (incongruent minus neutral trials) for both EF and CP immediately following stimulation (early block).

Source: Reprinted with permission from MIT Press: *Journal of Cognitive Neuroscience* (Esterman et al., 2006), © (2006).

Author commentary by Lynn C. Robertson

The ideas that led to the experiment came about indirectly, being motivated by more than 20 years of work with neurological patients with parietal lobe damage. Directly after receiving my doctorate in cognitive psychology, I accepted a postdoctoral position at a medical centre where I began attending rounds with neurologists and neuropsychologists. This was in the early 1980s and, at the time, perceptual problems that occurred when certain parts of the brain were damaged were of little interest to the vast majority of cognitive psychologists. When I described what I was observing on the neurology ward to my cognitive colleagues, most advised me to leave well alone. But I was too intrigued by the perceptual failures I was witnessing and found the challenges exhilarating. Thus began a long research career that includes unusual perceptual and attentional phenomena.

The seed for the current study was planted in this context in the late 1980s. My postdoctoral student Mirjam Eglin, a neurologist Robert Knight and I began studying visual search abilities in patients with unilateral neglect. Unilateral neglect is a deficit in spatially orienting attention and is generally associated with parietal damage to the human brain (including the inferior parietal lobe; see Chapter 4). The deficits in patients with neglect vary in severity and constellation of symptoms, but the common denominator is missing items on the side of space opposite to the damaged hemisphere (i.e. right hemisphere damage produces left neglect). In some patients, it appears as if one side of space disappears completely from conscious awareness. In other patients, information may be detected by a very slow, prodding search.

These symptoms are consistent with physiological results in animals that were just beginning to appear in the neurobiological literature in the early 1980s, suggesting two distinct visual pathways through the primate cortex; one originating in primary visual cortex, traversing dorsally through the parietal and frontal lobes that processed spatial information; and another originating in primary visual cortex traversing ventrally through the temporal lobe that processed object features (coined the 'where' and 'what' pathways, respectively).

Another line of evidence that appeared at about the same time was published in the cognitive literature, specifically the research reported by Anne Treisman that led to feature integration theory (FIT). In its original form FIT proposed that unique features such as colour, shape, motion, orientation, size, and so on were preattentively coded in separate 'feature maps', but in order to conjoin features from these different maps into bound units, spatial attention was required. A feature target (e.g. red circle) among a variable number of distractors (e.g. blue and green circles) popped out of the display; that is, reaction times to detect the presence or absence of the red circle were the same regardless of the number of distractors. Conversely, a target that required finding the conjunction of two features (e.g. red circle among red squares and blue circles) produced increasingly longer reaction times as the number of distractors increased. Attention was needed to find conjunctions but not to find features. Since patients with parietal lesions leading to unilateral neglect exhibit a severe spatial attention deficit, we hypothesized that conjunction search would be severely impacted on the contralesional side, while feature search would not.

This hypothesis was supported. Features on the 'neglected' side popped out, but conjunctions did not. We went on to replicate and extend these findings in other studies of unilateral neglect, but in the meantime a rare case of a patient with bilateral parietal damage emerged. Damage to both parietal lobes is fortunately very rare; as it leaves a person functionally blind, since spatial processing is disrupted across the entire visual field (neuropsychologically known as Balint's syndrome). Paradoxically, the visual information that is coded by the visual system continues to support perception of one object, but only one, at any given time. Patients with this type of damage have no control over where attentional allocation is directed or when an object they see will be replaced by another object in their perceptual experience. When we tested our patient in visual search studies, we again found that features popped out of a display but finding a conjunction was virtually impossible. We went on to link this problem with a feature binding deficit. We showed two differently coloured letters simultaneously on a computer screen and asked the patient to simply tell us which letter he saw and report its colour. He was nearly as likely to report the letter in the correct colour as in the colour of the other letter on the screen. He was quite certain about his report. The colours were bound randomly to the letters.

In 1982 Treisman and her colleagues had shown that these types of error, which she termed 'illusory conjunctions', could occur in normal perceivers when stimuli were shown for a fraction of a second and attention was diverted, but for our patient who could not move attention voluntarily, the display could be shown for up to 10 seconds, and illusory conjunctions were still present. We concluded that the attentional functions of the parietal lobes were critically involved in binding together features coded by specialized neural populations in the ventral pathway.

When I presented these findings at professional meetings, I was often asked if I would predict a type of 'hyperbinding' if the parietal lobes were overactive. I responded that if such a case existed, then yes, there should be more parietal activity. At the time, one of my students Noam Sagiv had become interested in synaesthesia, and it dawned on me that synaesthesia might be a case of 'hyperbinding'. This insight first led to several studies about the role attention might play in synaesthesia. Colour–grapheme synaesthesia was chosen as the exemplar because it was more closely tied to the feature binding deficits I had studied in patients. In a series of experiments Noam and I found that attention modulated the synaesthetic percept. When the inducing achromatic (e.g. grey) letter was outside the focus of attention, less synaesthesia resulted than when the letter was the focus of attention. Also, a review of the functional imaging literature on synaesthesia revealed that the inferior parietal lobe was active in almost every case. These two bits of information led to the hypothesis tested in the current paper; namely that the parietal lobe plays a role in binding synaesthetic colour and form.

Michael Esterman, a graduate student working in my laboratory, was conducting studies of attention, parietal activity and the binding problem, and he suggested that we use TMS to test the binding hypothesis of synaesthesia. This was a great idea, and we teamed up with Richard Ivry and Timothy Verstynen who were more knowledgeable about TMS to run the study. Fortunately, our hypothesis was supported.

The results of this study were particularly satisfying to me, since I had stuck my neck out in my 2003 *Nature Reviews* article on binding in which I used our findings on binding with patients and applied them to synaesthesia. Basically, the hypothesis we tested supported my predictions that were voiced in that paper. Although I am still not clear about how a shape produces a colour signal in the brain, it appears that once the colour signal has been generated, the neural network that supports normal colour/form binding is called into service to produce synaesthetic colour/form binding. A new student in my laboratory Bryan Alverez and I are now following up these findings.

I think this study is valuable because it shows that synaesthetic binding uses the same binding mechanisms as non-synaesthetic binding. It is important to note that synaesthetes perceive the wavelength colour of a letter as well as the synaesthetic colour. The main difference between non-synaesthetes and synaesthetes is that synaesthetes require two bindings (the colour induced by wavelength and the colour induced by form). In this sense the term 'hyperbinding' is not quite correct; rather, there is more binding required due to the extra colour signal, and when this occurs there will be more parietal activity.

When talking with others about synaesthesia (at least with those who are not synaesthetes), I am struck by the typical assumption that wavelength induced colour is somehow more real than synaesthetically induced colour. At the cortical level, a colour signal is a colour signal. The source of that signal is in the stimulus, but the signal itself must come from neurons that are involved in perception of colour. In colour-grapheme synaesthesia the source is a letter shape. Once the shape generates the colour, the solution for binding them together is the same.

I am encouraged by the increasing number of studies of synaesthesia appearing in the literature today, and I am invited to review more manuscripts on the subject than I can possibly accept. It is also exciting to work on a phenomenon that seems intractable on the surface and to have contributed to making it scientifically tractable. My experimental work with patients and with synaesthetes have been both challenging but tremendously rewarding in this regard.

Author commentary by John J. Foxe

I first learned of synaesthesia[2] from Professor Peter Grossenbacher[3] back in the early 1990s. He was at that time one of less than a handful of brave souls that I knew to be active in synaesthesia research, which was considered a decidedly esoteric, and truth be told, rather dubious topic of study for a 'serious' neuroscientist to be mixed up in back then. In fact, I recall many conferences and presentations where there were heated arguments as to the very existence of the condition, and there were more than a few who suspected that malingering was at the nub of it. It is remarkable and gratifying to have witnessed the extent to which things have transformed over the intervening years. This early work by Peter, Professor Robertson's group of course, and the many others who took up the challenge in the interim, has established synaesthesia as a condition very much worthy of study. In any case, something Peter said back then about synaesthesia has resonated with me since. I recall an occasion at the annual conference of the International Multisensory Research Forum (IMRF) in New York in 2001, when an audience member asked him whether his interest in this extremely rare condition, as it was then thought to be, was because he himself was a synaesthete. His retort was that he was lamentably 'only a wannabe synaesthete'. 'Why'?, one might ask. But it turns out that this is not such a curious stance. As I have found myself describing synaesthesia to non-scientist friends, and the occasional unfortunate who was foolish enough to ask me what I do for a living, I have been surprised at the number of folk who have expressed sentiments similar to Peter's.

There appears to be a common feeling that there is a richness of experience in synaesthetic perception that might well be life enriching. I am put in mind of a favourite childhood film, *The Wizard of Oz*, with the bleak greyness of Kansas giving way to the technicoloured experience of Oz for Dorothy and her companions. Some years later, the notion that synaesthesia might confer special powers on its 'sufferers' was confirmed for me when I read Joseph Gleick's (1992) truly superb biography of the great physicist Richard Feynman – *Genius*. There is a wonderful passage where Feynman is doing his best to explain how he can hold onto the various facets of a complex problem or equation and he explains that 'Lambda is brown of course' and then in exasperation, he gripes that students will never be able to understand all of this. The reference to colour-grapheme associations is not explicitly remarked on by Gleick, who appears not to realize the significance, but it seemed clear to me that Feynman must in fact have been a synaesthete and that he was able to put this extra dimensionality of experience to very good use in his calculations. Given my own rather severe mathematical limitations, a real burden for somebody trying to work in the neurosciences, I have had cause over the years to echo Peter Grossenbacher's wish, as I too find myself a 'wannabe synaesthete'.

It is a great pleasure and privilege for me to have the opportunity to write about the work of Professor Lynn Robertson and her group on synaesthesia and attention. I have followed Lynn's opus with admiration and keen interest for many years now. Her work on feature integration has left little doubt that spatial attention mechanisms, subserved in great part by cortical regions in the right posterior parietal lobe, play a crucial role in the so-called binding problem. It would be difficult to overstate the importance of this insight, which builds on the ground-breaking work of Professor Anne Treisman and her influential feature integration theory (FIT) of attention. The details of the findings in the Easterman paper have been most ably described by Professors Roche and Commins above, and so I will not belabour them here. As with any well-crafted study, the Easterman paper raises as many provocative questions as it answers, and it is to these questions that I will devote the rest of this commentary. The first thing to note of course is that the Robertson group's interest in conducting this beautifully executed TMS study was not so much about understanding synaesthesia as it was about leveraging this curious condition as a means to understand 'normal' human attentional functions. Nonetheless, the results also have important implications for models of synaesthesia, and as we will come to below, raise questions about some of the rather simplistic notions that still dominate current thinking about this condition.

Various models have been proposed to account for synaesthesia with the common thread being the concept of over-exuberant anatomical connectivity giving rise to anomalous cross-activation of one cortical region by another (e.g. Grossenbacher and Lovelace, 2001; Smilek et al., 2001). In most of these conceptions, the implication is that the connectivity and resulting communication between these areas is a direct affair. In the case of colour-grapheme synaesthesia, the thinking is that the so-called visual word form area (VWFA) must have a surfeit of lateral connections with the closely neighbouring colour-processing area (V4). The VWFA is thought to occupy a tract of cortex in the left mid-fusiform gyrus (e.g. Cohen et al., 2000) and human V4 lies along the lingual gyrus and may extend onto the fusiform gyrus (e.g. Gallant et al., 2000).

Recent anatomical imaging data has indeed pointed to structural differences in this general region in synaesthesia (Rouw and Scholte, 2007). The clear implication then is that illusory synaesthetic conjunctions of the colour-grapheme variety are actually a function of local connections between these two areas, most likely constitutively active. Thus, according to the over-exuberance model, for want of a better moniker, it would have to be considered quite puzzling that a control region in the parietal lobes could intervene in this 'local' cross-coupling. Now I would be remiss if I did not also mention that the very existence of a VWFA has been vigorously questioned (see Price and Devlin, 2003), as if things needed more complicating. These authors have shown that the area identified as the VWFA is also activated by a large assortment of non-word stimulus types and tasks requiring no orthographic processing, and most damagingly for the over-exuberance hypothesis, the VWFA has even been shown to be active during a colour-naming task (Price et al., 1996). It hardly needs pointing out that if there is a common region for both colour and word form processing, then the inter-regional cross-connectivity notion may need some rethinking.

In a similar vein, how are we to reconcile the intriguing findings of Easterman and Robertson with the results from neuroimaging investigations of colour-grapheme synaesthetes (e.g. Hubbard et al., 2005)? If the colour is not bound to the grapheme when the right parietal region is taken off-line, then what of the fMRI studies that have shown cross-activation within these ventral visual areas? One explanation may lie in the temporal resolution of hemodynamic imaging. That is, since fMRI measurements of the haemodynamic response amount to an integration of activity over a very long time period, simply because a measure of the brain's plumbing, which is essentially what fMRI amounts to, is by definition a measure of a very sluggish response. Thus, the technique cannot distinguish early feedforward from later feedback processes. As such, it is entirely possible that the ventral activity seen in these studies occurs subsequent to initial binding mechanisms within higher-order attentional control regions of the parietal lobe. Indeed, it could just as easily represent late post-perceptual imagery of the illusory conjunctions as earlier perceptual processes.

Another point to note is that synaesthesia comes in two obviously different forms, the far more common form being within a sensory modality, like the colour-grapheme synaesthesia investigated in the Easterman paper. Note that there is a tendency for this to be referred to as a multisensory phenomenon, but it is not since the bound features are both visual. The second major form is the true multisensory variety where perceptions are linked between sensory systems and these conjunctions can be some of the most exotic found in synaesthesia. One famous case, for example, was presented by the neurologist Richard Cytowic who in 1993 described the extraordinary case of a man who tasted shapes (Cytowic, 1993 [2003]), and in so doing was responsible for a huge upsurge in the interest in synaesthesia. In any case, the intrasensory variety is by far the more common, whereas the cross-sensory or multisensory variety is considerably more rare, although it does appear to be relatively more common in professional musicians, which may not come as such a surprise. The fact that the former variety is far more common than the latter lends itself nicely to the over-exuberance model, suggesting once again that this may be a cortical geographic issue. Intrasensory cross talk would necessarily rely on over-exuberant communication between relatively closely neighbouring cortical regions as detailed above, and so it is relatively intuitive to think that some surplus of short-range direct connections might have developed.

On the other hand, if multisensory synaesthesia also relies on aberrant connections, then its relative rarity could be due to the large distance between the respective cortical regions, which is measured in centimetres rather than at the millimetre scale. However, there is a potential problem with this latter line of reasoning also, despite its obvious intuitive appeal. Over the last 10 years, it has emerged that the sensory systems are not nearly as anatomically isolated from each other as was originally thought. Anatomic tracer studies have found that there is far more cross-connectivity at nearly every hierarchical level between the various sensory systems, including between the initial primary sensory regions of the visual and auditory systems (e.g. Falchier et al., 2002; Rockland and Ojima, 2003).

In light of this, it is worth introducing a very recent study by Professor Michael Beauchamp of The University of Texas and my colleague at City College, New York (CCNY), Professor Tony Ro (Beauchamp and Ro, 2008). This study is highly instructive regarding the issue of connectivity in synaesthesia in my view. They studied a single neurological patient, who subsequent to a localized lesion in the thalamus developed a strong auditory-tactile synaesthesia, whereby the patient experienced strong tactile tingling sensations in response to certain specific sounds. Using fMRI, Michael and Tony found that secondary somatosensory cortex was strongly activated in this patient in response to sounds that induced the synaesthetic tinglings; a pattern that was not evoked by non-inducing sounds, and a pattern that was entirely absent in a group of healthy control subjects. Their interpretation of these results is in line with the over-exuberance hypothesis in that they attributed the emergence of the synaesthesia to 'abnormal connections between sensory modalities that are normally separate' and 'inappropriate connections between nearby cortical territories'. Their thesis was that since the thalamic lesion had resulted in a loss of somatosensory inputs, new connections had developed. It is on this point that I would have to disagree with my colleagues. First, it is now well established that connections between the auditory and somatosensory systems are much more extensive than was once thought and that there are hierarchically early regions of both auditory and somatosensory cortex that are responsive to both auditory and tactile inputs (see e.g. Schroeder and Foxe, 2002; Foxe and Schroeder, 2005).

As above, the same is true for auditory-visual connections (e.g. Falchier et al., 2002). It seems highly unlikely to me that new and inappropriate connections develop between neighbouring regions in an adult brain. Rather, a more likely scenario is that already present but relatively latent inputs to these are unmasked when direct afferent input from the primary sense is removed. In the majority of healthy humans, one suspects that these latent cross-connections serve a modulatory function allowing for a level of binding that does not reach awareness but is nonetheless crucial for normal object formation. In the case of synaesthesia, these normal latent inputs may be overactive, or in keeping with the over-exuberance hypothesis, perhaps there are simply rather more of them than in the typical brain. The answer to this issue is unlikely in my view to be answerable at the level of non-invasive structural anatomy measures with MRI and it may take careful post-mortem stereologic procedures to adequately address the question.

There is another point that surely needs to be made about the Easterman study. One conspicuous issue with applying the feature integration notion to synaesthesia remains the fact that in colour-grapheme synaesthesia, there is no need for the actual colour to be present at all. That is, gray or black letters induce the colour percepts. As such, there is no other feature in the retinal image to be bound and the achromatic shapes of the letters somehow induce this other illusory feature. And so, while the fact that TMS can 'unbind' these shape–colour associations is truly intriguing, it remains difficult for me at least to fully conceptualize what is being bound in the first place. Regardless, the Easterman study is clear that something is indeed being unbound.

I finish by mentioning a study from our own work that was conducted at Trinity College in Dublin in the lab of Professor Fiona Newell. We took a rather different approach in this study in that we decided not to try to look at orthographic stimuli at all in our colour-grapheme synaesthetes. Instead, using high-density event-related potential (ERP) recordings, we simply asked if there were basic sensory processing differences early in the visual system in a large cohort of synaesthetes. Unlike the temporal resolution issues with fMRI pointed out above, the ERP technique allows us to assess sensory and perceptual processing at the millisecond scale. A full exposition of the results is not possible or warranted here but the main finding is certainly germane. We found clear evidence of very early differences in visual sensory processing that began just 70–100 msec after stimulus presentation, which is only about 25–30 msec after initial afference in the primary visual cortex in response to simple visual stimuli that did not induce synaesthetic experiences (Barnett et al., 2008b).

So, our data too suggest a basic difference in the wiring of the synaesthetic brain, a difference that impacts very early sensory processing. The plot thickens and much work remains to be done. How are we to resolve such early differences that suggest bottom-up feed-forward processes with the evidence from Easterman that top-down attentional control regions can affect this processing? Is there enough time for these regions to exert such control? As with any great experiment, the Easterman paper presented and continues to pose a real challenge for the field, and in doing so, it has advanced our knowledge in no small way.

Notes

1   There has been difficulty in assessing the true prevalence of synaesthesia in the population due to the presence of a self-selection bias in those who report the experience; estimates of prevalence range from 1 in 20 to 1 in 2,000.
2   Synaesthesia is from Greek – syn meaning 'plus' or 'union' and aesthesis meaning 'sensation'.
3   Peter is now at Naropa University in Colorado.

References

Barnett, K.J., Finucane, C., Asher, J.E. et al. (2008a) Familial patterns and the origins of individual differences in synaesthesia, *Cognition*, 106(2): 871–93.

Barnett, K.J., Foxe, J.J., Molholm, S. et al. (2008b) Differences in early sensory-perceptual processing in synesthesia: a visual evoked potentials study, *Neuroimage*, 43: 605–13.

Beauchamp, M.S. and Ro, T. (2008) Neural substrates of sound-touch synesthesia after a thalamic lesion, *Journal of Neuroscience*, 28(50): 13696–702.

Cohen, L., Dehaene, S., Naccache, L. et al. (2000) The visual word form area: spatial and temporal characterization of an initial stage of reading in normal subjects and posterior split-brain patients, *Brain*, 123(2): 291–307.

Cytowic, R.E. (1993 [2003]) *The Man Who Tasted Shapes*. New York: Putnam.

Donner, T.H., Kettermann, A., Diesch, E. et al. (2002) Visual feature and conjunction searches of equal difficulty engage only partially overlapping frontoparietal networks, *NeuroImage*, 15: 16–25.

Falchier, A., Clavagnier, S., Barone, P. and Kennedy, H. (2002) Anatomical evidence of multimodal integration in primate striate cortex, *Journal of Neuroscience*, 22(13): 5749–59.

Foxe, J.J. and Schroeder, C.E. (2005) The case for feedforward multisensory convergence during early cortical processing, *Neuroreport*, 16(5): 419–23.

Gallant, J.L., Shoup, R.E. and Mazer, J.A. (2000) A human extrastriate area functionally homologous to macaque V4, *Neuron*, 27(2): 227–35.

Gleick, J. (1992) *Genius: The Life and Science of Richard Feynman*. New York: Pantheon Books.

Grossenbacher, P.G. and Lovelace, C.T. (2001) Mechanisms of synaesthesia: cognitive and physiological constraints, *Trends in Cognitive Sciences*, 5: 36–41.

Hubbard, E.M., Arman, A.C., Ramachandran, V.S. and Boynton, G.M. (2005) Individual differences among grapheme-colour synaesthetes: brain-behavior correlations, *Neuron*, 45: 975–85.

Price, C.J. and Devlin, J.T. (2003) The myth of the visual word form area, *Neuroimage*, 19(3): 473–81.

Price, C.J., Moore, C.J., Humphreys, G.W., Frackowiak, R.S. and Friston, K.J. (1996) The neural regions sustaining object recognition and naming. *Proceedings of the Biological Society*, 263(1376): 1501–7.

Rockland, K.S. and Ojima, H. (2003) Multisensory convergence in calcarine visual areas in macaque monkey, *International Journal of Psychophysiology*, 50(1–2): 19–26.

Rouw, R. and Scholte, H.S. (2007) Increased structural connectivity in grapheme-color synesthesia, *Nature Neuroscience*, 10(6): 792–7.

Schroeder, C.E. and Foxe, J.J. (2002) The timing and laminar profile of converging inputs to multisensory areas of the macaque neocortex, *Brain Research: Cognitive Brain Research*, 14(1): 187–98.

Smilek, D., Dixon, M.J., Cudahy, C. and Merikle, P.M. (2001) Synaesthetic photisms influence visual perception, *Journal of Cognitive Neuroscience*, 13: 930.

Sperling, J.M., Prvulovic, D., Linden, D.E., Singer, W. and Stirn, A. (2006) Neuronal correlates of colour-graphemic synaesthesia: a fMRI study, *Cortex*, 42(2): 295–303.

Walsh, V. and Pascual-Leone, A. (2003) *Transcranial Magnetic Stimulation: A Neurochronometrics of Mind*. Cambridge, MA: MIT Press.

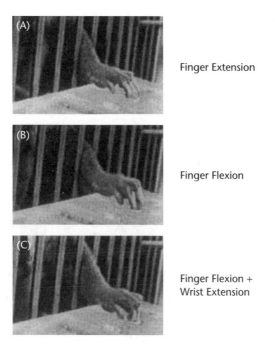

Finger Extension

Finger Flexion

Finger Flexion +
Wrist Extension

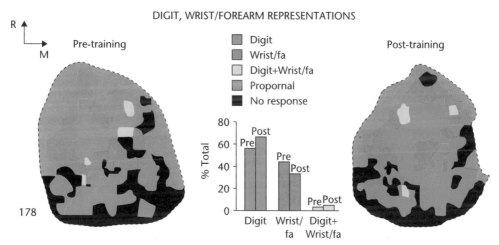

DIGIT, WRIST/FOREARM REPRESENTATIONS

R

M

Pre-training

Post-training

Digit
Wrist/fa
Digit+Wrist/fa
Propornal
No response

% Total

Post
Pre

Pre
Post

Pre Post

Digit   Wrist/   Digit+
         fa   Wrist/fa

178

Figure 2.2 (Top) Sequence of photographs showing movements used to retrieve food from a well of a Khiver board. (A) the fingers extended as the arm moved towards the well. (B) the fingers flexed within the well and then stopped. (C) a second finger flexion occurred, but before the finger flexion movement was completed the wrist extended. (Bottom) Representation of the distal forelimb in cortical area 4 derived from pre- and post-training mapping procedures in three training animals.

Source: Nudo, R.J., Milliken, G.W., Jenkins, W.M., Merzenich, M.M. Use-dependent alterations of movement representations in primary motor cortex of adult squirrel monkeys. Journal of Neuroscience. 1996 Jan 15;16(2): 785–807.

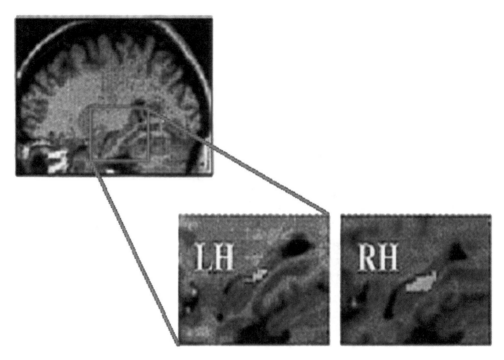

Figure 7.1 (Top) Sagittal section of an MRI scan with the hippocampus indicated by the box. (Bottom) Group results superimposed onto the scan of an individual subject selected at random. Increased grey matter volume in the posterior of the left and right hippocampi (LH and RH, respectively) of taxi drivers relative to those of controls.

Source: Reprinted with permission from the National Academy of Science: *PNAS* (Maguire et al., 2000), © (2000).

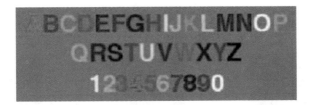

Figure 8.1 Synaesthetic alphabet for participant EF.

Source: Reprinted with permission from MIT Press: *Journal of Cognitive Neuroscience* (Esterman et al., 2006), © (2006).

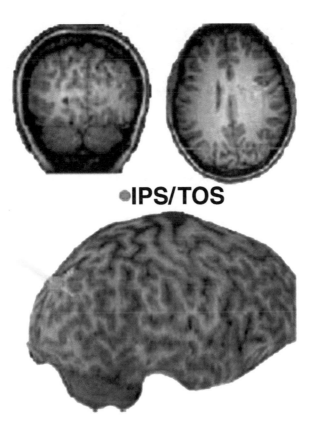

Figure 8.2 Target stimulation site (right IPS/TOS) shown on coronal and axial slices, plus a 3-D reconstruction of the anatomical image for EF. Target location is shown in red, centre of magnetic coil is shown as green spheres in the 3-D image, and estimated pulse and orthogonal trajectories are shown as yellow lines.

Source: Reprinted with permission from MIT Press: *Journal of Cognitive Neuroscience* (Esterman et al., 2006), © (2006).

Congruent   Incongruent   Neutral

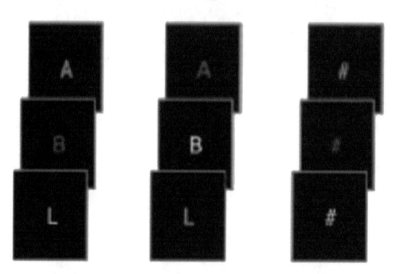

Figure 8.3 Individualized experimental conditions. The task was to name the stimulus colour. In the congruent condition, the stimulus colour matched the synaesthetic colour. In the incongruent condition, the stimulus colour did not match the synaesthetic colour. Neutral characters did not evoke a synaesthetic colour.

Source: Reprinted with permission from MIT Press: *Journal of Cognitive Neuroscience* (Esterman et al., 2006), © (2006).

Appendices

Appendix 1 – Chapter 2

Modulation of Muscle Responses Evoked by Transcranial Magnetic Stimulation During the Acquisition of New Fine Motor Skills

Pascual-Leone, A., Nguyet, D., Cohen, L.G., Brasil-Neto, J.P., Cammarota, A. and Hallett, M. (1995)
Journal of Neurophysiology, 74(3): 1037–45.

Summary and conclusions

1. We used transcranial magnetic stimulation (TMS) to study the role of plastic changes of the human motor system in the acquisition of new fine motor skills. We mapped the cortical motor areas targeting the contralateral long finger flexor and extensor muscles in subjects learning a one-handed, five-finger exercise on the piano. In a second experiment, we studied the different effects of mental and physical practice of the same five-finger exercise on the modulation of the cortical motor areas targeting muscles involved in the task.

2. Over the course of 5 days, as subjects learned the one-handed, five-finger exercise through daily 2-h manual practice sessions, the cortical motor areas targeting the long finger flexor and extensor muscles enlarged, and their activation threshold decreased. Such changes were limited to the cortical representation of the hand used in the exercise. No changes of cortical motor outputs occurred in control subjects who underwent daily TMS mapping but did not practice on the piano at all (*control group 1*).

3. We studied the effect of increased hand use without specific skill learning in subjects who played the piano at will for 2 h each day using only the right hand but who were not taught the five-finger exercise (*control group 2*) and who did not practice any specific task. In these control subjects, the changes in cortical motor outputs were similar but significantly less prominent than in those occurring in the test subjects, who learned the new skill.

4. In the second experiment, subjects were randomly assigned to a physical practice group, a mental practice group, or a control group. Subjects in each practice group physically or mentally practiced the five-finger piano exercise independently for 2 h daily for 5 days. The control group did not practice the exercise. All subjects had daily TMS mapping of the cortical motor areas targeting the long finger flexor and extensor muscles.

5. Over the course of 5 days, mental practice alone led to significant improvement in the performance of the five-finger exercise, but the improvement was significantly less than that produced by physical practice alone. However, mental

practice alone led to the same plastic changes in the motor system as those occurring with the acquisition of the skill by repeated physical practice.

6. We conclude that acquisition of the motor skills needed for the correct performance of a five-finger piano exercise is associated with modulation of the cortical motor outputs to the muscles involved in the task. This rapid modulation may occur through an increase of synaptic efficacy in existing neural circuits (long-term potentiation) or unmasking of existing connections due to disinhibition.

7. Mental practice alone seems to be sufficient to promote the modulation of neural circuits involved in the early stages of motor skill learning. This modulation not only results in marked performance improvement but also seems to place the subjects at an advantage for further skill learning with minimal physical practice.

Introduction

Playing the piano demands orderly, sequential control of individual finger movements and a high degree of bimanual coordination. Even when given information about the hand position, the finger motions, the sequence of keys to press, and the duration and velocity of each key press, a novice would still be unable to play even the simplest piano sonata. The piano student must understand the demands of the task, develop a cognitive representation of it, and initiate a first, centrally guided response. At first, his or her limbs will move slowly, with fluctuating accuracy and speed, and success will require visual, proprioceptive, and auditory feedback. With practice, the pianist can refine each single movement, link the different movements with the desired timing, and attain stability and fluency in the ordered sequence. Only then can the pianist shift his or her attention from the mechanical details of the performance to its artistic interpretation.

Acquisition of new fine motor skills may demand modification of the nervous system to accommodate the new procedures (Jenkins et al., 1990; Kaas 1991; Merzenich et al., 1990). The primary motor cortex (M1) may have a central role in skill learning considering the flexibility in the associations of sensory inputs to M1 neurons and in the associations between M1, spinal neurons, and somatic musculature (Aou et al., 1992; Iriki et al., 1989; Kaas 1991). Studies using noninvasive imaging and neurophysiological techniques have demonstrated skill-associated nervous system plasticity in humans. In blind subjects, for example, proficient Braille reading is associated with enlargement of the cortical sensorimotor representation of the reading finger (Pascual-Leone et al., 1993; Pascual-Leone and Torres 1993), and in normal subjects, learning of a complicated sequence of voluntary finger movements is associated with changes in the slow cortical DC potentials (Niemann et al., 1991) and transient increases in regional cerebral blood flow in the cerebellum and striatum (Seitz et al., 1990).

In the present study we used transcranial magnetic stimulation (TMS) to study the cortical motor areas targeting the contralateral long finger flexor and extensor muscles in subjects learning a one-handed, five-finger exercise on the piano. In a second experiment we studied the different effects of mental and physical practice on the acquisition of the same five-finger exercise and on the modulation of the cortical motor areas targeting muscles involved in the task.

Methods

Subjects

We used different subjects for each experiment. In *experiment 1*, we studied 18 subjects who were randomly assigned to a test group or one of two control groups. Each group consisted of three men and three women who were matched for age (mean age, 44 yr; range, 38–51 yr). In *experiment 2*, we studied 15 subjects who were randomly assigned to a physical practice group, a mental practice group, or a control group. Each group consisted of three men and two women who were matched for age (mean age, 32 yr; range, 19–42 yr). All subjects were right-handed, as determined by the Oldfield questionnaire (Oldfield 1971). None of the subjects had experience playing the piano or any other musical instrument. None of them knew how to typewrite using all fingers. None of them had jobs or were involved in daily activities that demanded skilled, fine-finger movements. All subjects had normal findings on neurological and general physical examinations. The protocol was approved by the Institutional Review Board, and all subjects gave their written informed consent for the study. The transcranial magnetic stimulator was used under an Investigational Device Exemption from the Food and Drug Administration.

Experiment 1

In *experiment 1*, subjects performed the one-handed, five-finger exercise on a Yamaha electronic piano keyboard interfaced with a Macintosh IIci computer. The exercise consisted of the following sequence of finger movements (and notes): thumb (C), index finger (D), middle finger (E), ring finger (F), little finger (G), ring finger (F), middle finger (E), index finger (D). A metronome marked a rhythm of 60 beats per minute, and the subjects were asked to match the thumb and little finger movements to the beat, intercalating the movements of the other fingers between the beats. The subjects were asked to try to perform the sequence of finger movements fluently, without pauses, and without skipping any key, and to pay particular attention to keeping the interval between the individual key presses constant and the duration and velocity of each key press the same.

On *day 1*, baseline TMS mapping of the cortical motor areas targeting the long finger flexor and extensor muscles bilaterally was done according to the technique described below. Subjects were then randomly assigned to a test group or to one of two control groups. Only subjects in the test group were taught the five-finger exercise. Thereafter, they practiced the exercise for 2 h daily on *days 1–5*, had their performance tested, rested for 20–30 min, and had TMS mapping of the motor cortex.

The performance was tested by recording 20 sequential repetitions of the exercise on the computer with the use of a sequencing software package (Vision, Opcode, Menlo Park, CA) that allowed the analysis of the exact sequence of key presses, the interval between key presses, and the duration and velocity of each key press. Any key pressed out of order was considered an error, so more than one error was possible during each sequence. The anticipated interval between key presses was 0.25 s given that a rhythm of 60 beats per minute was marked by a metronome for each four intervals. After each daily test, the subjects were given feedback about their performance, as well as tips on how to improve.

Control group 1 had daily TMS mapping only. *Control group 2* played the piano at will for 2 h each day with the use of only the right hand, rested for 20–30 min, and had daily TMS mapping. Subjects in *control group 2* could play anything they wanted on the piano but were asked to press only one key at a time, therefore executing individual finger movements in self-generated sequences. They were asked not to repeat a given sequence. On *day 5, control groups 1* and *2* were also taught the exercise, and their performance on the test was recorded as for the test subjects.

All practice sessions were performed in the laboratory and were supervised by one of the investigators. Subjects were asked not to rehearse the task at home.

Experiment 2

In *experiment 2*, all subjects were taught the same five-finger exercise as in *experiment 1*. Baseline TMS mapping of their cortical motor areas targeting the long finger flexor and extensor muscles was done according to the technique described below. Thereafter, the subjects were randomly assigned to a physical practice group, a mental practice group, or a control group.

Subjects in each practice group physically or mentally practiced the exercise independently for 2 h daily for 5 days. The control group did not practice the exercise but had daily TMS mapping. Subjects were asked not to rehearse the task at home. During the practice session, subjects in the physical practice group were encouraged to repeatedly perform the exercise on the keyboard and were free to select their own strategy. Subjects in the mental practice group were asked to sit in front of the piano and try to visualize their fingers performing the exercise and to imagine the sound. They were not allowed to touch the piano keys or to rehearse the exercise by moving the fingers in the air. To assure that they were indeed not moving their fingers, electromyographic (EMG) activity from the long finger flexor and extensor muscles was monitored continually with the use of pairs of surface EMG electrodes taped to the skin over the belly of the muscle and displaying the activity on an oscilloscope at a sensitivity of 20 μV/div. After the 1st 10–15 min, all subjects were able to follow the instructions without difficulty. The mental practice group had a single 2-h physical practice session at the end of *day 5*. The results of task performance and TMS mapping following this physical practice session are reported as *day 5'*.

The performance of all subjects was tested daily by 20 sequential repetitions of the exercise in the same fashion as described for *experiment 1*. TMS mapping was performed 20–30 min after the test. Therefore performance assessment and TMS mapping were the same in all three groups, which differed only in the learning conditions.

Transcranial magnetic stimulation and mapping technique

We used a Cadwell MES-10 magnetic stimulator equipped with an 8-shaped coil, which was held flat on the scalp with the intersection of its two 'wings' centered over a defined scalp position; the handle of the coil was held horizontally, tangentially to the subject's head, pointing occipitally. This technique allows relatively focal stimulation (Cohen et al., 1990; Maccabee et al., 1990). The brain structures stimulated might be inferred from models of the induced electric fields (Roth et al., 1991a,b; Tofts 1990). However, this approximation might be affected by the existence of bends in the course of fibers that lower their threshold (Maccabee et al., 1993). In any case, overlay of TMS maps onto the magnetic resonance image of the subject's brain suggests that the motor responses are evoked from activation of the primary motor cortex (Levy et al., 1991; Wassermann et al., 1992).

For cortical mapping, scalp positions 1 cm apart were stimulated successively, following the technique described by Wassermann et al. (1991), and we calculated contour maps of the probability of evoking a motor potential with a peak-to-peak amplitude of at least 50 μV in the contralateral muscles according to the stimulated scalp position. Eight single stimuli were given at each scalp position. On average, a stimulus was delivered every 3–5 s. Each contour map represents 25 scalp positions (1 cm apart) arranged in a 5×5 grid around the 'optimal' scalp position, which was marked on the subject's scalp with indelible ink. The mark, which remained throughout the 5-day experiment, was used as a reference point for the daily mapping. The optimal scalp position was the one from which TMS elicited motor evoked potentials (MEPs) of maximal amplitude in the contralateral finger flexor or extensor muscles. We have previously shown that optimal scalp positions determined in this manner project onto the posterior bank of the precentral sulcus and seem to represent activation of the primary motor cortex (Wassermann et al., 1992). The stimulus intensity was 110 per cent of the subject's threshold on each particular day. Motor threshold was defined by the method of limits. In each subject we determined threshold as the average result from six series of stimuli, three with ascending stimulation intensities and three with descending stimulation intensities. The order of these six series of stimuli was randomly varied across subjects. For the ascending series we began stimulation at an intensity at which TMS did not evoke any identifiable MEPs in 10 trials. Thereafter, we increased the stimulation intensity in steps of 1 per cent of the stimulator output. At each new intensity we applied 10 stimuli. Threshold intensity was defined as the lowest stimulation intensity at which TMS evoked ≥ 5 MEPs of ≥ 50-μV peak-to-peak amplitude. For the descending series we first stimulated at an intensity at which TMS evoked MEPs of ≥ 50 μV peak-to-peak amplitude in 10 of 10 trials. Thereafter, we decreased the stimulation intensity in steps of 1 per cent of the stimulator output. At each new intensity we applied 10 stimuli. Threshold intensity was defined as the lowest stimulation intensity at which TMS evoked ≥ 5 MEPs of ≥ 50-μV peak-to-peak amplitude. Therefore the threshold in any given session represents the average value from six separate determinations and expresses the lowest stimulus intensity that evoked from the optimal scalp position motor potentials with a peak-to-peak amplitude of at least 50 μV in ≥ 50 per cent of the trials.

Mapping was performed with the subjects at rest. The absence of spontaneous, background EMG activity was documented by continuous EMG monitoring that was presented to the subjects by loudspeaker and on an oscilloscope at 20 μV per division. Subjects were instructed to relax the target muscles completely achieving auditory silence and a flat line on the oscilloscope. EMG activity was recorded with a Dantec Counterpoint electromyograph with the use of pairs of surface EMG electrodes taped to the skin over the belly of the superficial finger flexor and extensor muscles in the forearm. This recording setup was not selective for movements of any particular digit but rather allowed monitoring of flexion-extension activity of all fingers.

In both experiments the experimenter performing the TMS mapping was unaware of the group to which a given subject belonged in order to avoid biasing of the results.

Results

Experiment 1

Over the course of the 5 days, the test group's playing skill improved markedly (Figures 1 and 2). By *day 5*, the number of errors in the sequence of key presses clearly decreased, and the subjects correctly completed at least 18 of the 20 sequential repetitions of the exercise. The variability of the interval between key presses decreased, as illustrated by the narrowing of the standard deviation. The improvement in accuracy is illustrated by the decrease in the mean interval between key presses to 0.25 s, which corresponds with the interval specified by the rhythm of 60 beats per minute marked by the metronome.

Concurrently with this improvement in performance, the threshold for activation of the finger flexor and extensor muscles contralateral to the side of TMS decreased steadily over the course of the 5 days, but only for the hand being trained. In addition,

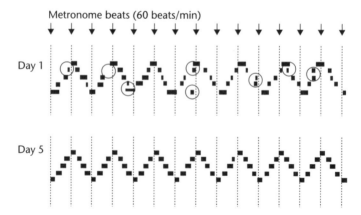

Figure 1 *Experiment 1*: example of the performance in the 5-finger exercise on *days 1* and 5 in a representative test subject. Arrows and dashed lines mark the metronome beats. Bars illustrate the different notes (finger movements) with the thumb being the lowest row of bars and the little finger the highest. The length of the bar represents the duration of each key press. Circles highlight the errors in the sequence performance. Comparison between *days 1* and 5 illustrate the large number of errors, the highly variable key press durations, and the frequent deviations from the metronome on *day 1*.

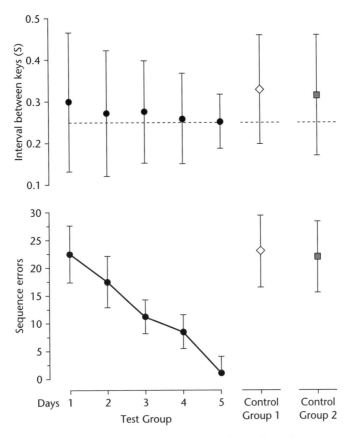

Figure 2 *Experiment 1*: inlerval between key presses and number of sequence errors for all subjects (mean ± SD) in the 20-sequence test (5-finger piano exercise) over the course of 5 days' learning. Dashed line indicates the anticipated interval of 0.25 s between key presses (see text for details).

the size of the cortical output map for both muscle groups increased (Figures 3 and 4). The increase in the size of the maps was independent of the threshold changes, because daily mapping of each muscle was performed at 110 per cent of the subject's threshold on that day, thus controlling the effects of threshold changes across days.

As predicted, skill learning did not take place in the control subjects. *Control groups 1 and 2* performed the exercise on *day 5* with the same accuracy as the test subjects on *day 1* (Figure 2). In *control group 1*, daily motor mapping with TMS did not affect the threshold for activation of the finger flexor and extensor muscles or the size of their cortical representation (Figure 4). In *control group 2*, increased daily use of the hand by random piano playing resulted in a slight decrease in the threshold for TMS activation of the finger flexor and extensor muscles and in some increase in the size of the cortical representation for both muscle groups (Figures 3 and 4). However, these changes were significantly smaller [$P < 0.001$, analysis of variance (ANOVA)] than in the test subjects.

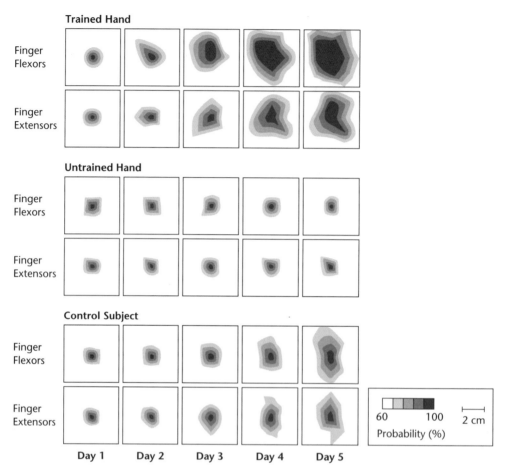

Figure 3 *Experiment 1*: representative examples of the cortical motor output maps for the long finger flexor and extensor musles on *days 1–5* in a test subject (trained and untrained hand) and a subject from *control group 2*. Each map is based on 25 measured points.

Experiment 2

Over the course of 5 days, both practice groups showed progressive improvement in their playing skills, as illustrated by a decrease in the number of sequence errors and a reduction in the variability (standard deviation) of the interval between key presses (Figure 5). Accuracy increased in all practice subjects, as illustrated by a decrease in the mean interval between key presses to 0.25 s. However, the physical practice group showed a significantly greater reduction ($P < 0.001$, ANOVA) in the number of sequence errors and a trend toward greater accuracy than did the mental practice group. The control group's performance did not improve.

Concurrently with the improvement in performance, the threshold for activation of the finger flexor and extensor muscles by TMS to the contralateral scalp decreased

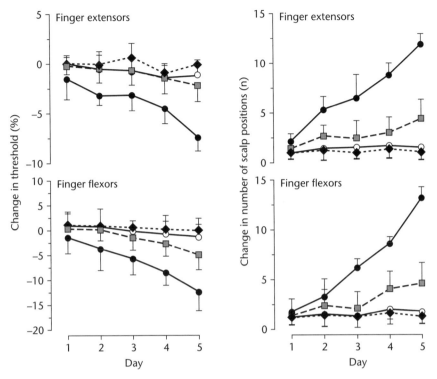

Figure 4 *Experiment 1*: change in motor threshold, expressed as a percentage of change from baseline threshold, and in number of scalp positions on the stimulation grid from which motor evoked potentials (MEPs) could be produced in the finger flexor and extensor muscles with a probability of ≥60 per cent in all subjects over the course of 5 days. Values are given as means ± SD. Filled circles, trained hand of test subjects; open circles, untrained hand of test subjects; filled diamonds, *control group 1*; stippled squares, *control group 2*.

steadily over the course of the 5 days in the physical and mental practice groups. In addition, even though the threshold decrease was taken into account, the size of the cortical representation for both muscle groups increased equally for both practice groups but did not increase for the control group (Figures 6 and 7).

Therefore mental practice alone led to significant fine motor skill learning but did not result in as much performance improvement as physical practice alone. However, mental practice alone led to the same plastic changes in the motor system as those occurring with the acquisition of a skill by repeated physical practice. By the end of *day 5*, the changes in the cortical motor outputs to the muscles involved in the task did not differ between the physical and the mental practice groups (Figure 5). However, the mental practice group's performance was at the level of that occurring with only 3 days' physical practice. After a single 2-h physical practice session, the mental practice group's performance improved to the level of 5 days' physical practice (Figure 5).

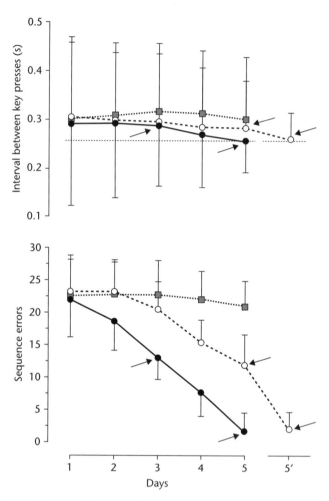

Figure 5 *Experiment 2*: interval between key presses and number of sequence errors for all subjects (mean ± SD) in the 20-sequence test (5-finger piano exercise) over the course of 5 days' learning. Dashed line indicates the anticipated interval between key presses (0.25 s). Arrows indicate the level of performance between the physical and mental practice groups at the end of *day 5* or *day 5′* (see text for details). Filled circles, physical practice group; open circles, mental practice group; stippled squares, control group; stippled circle, mental practice group on *day 5′*.

Discussion

Neurophysiological correlates of motor skill acquisition

Recently, studies using noninvasive neurophysiological and imaging techniques have suggested that even the adult human nervous system is capable of reorganizing after injury, with the probable purpose of minimizing deficits and producing recovery

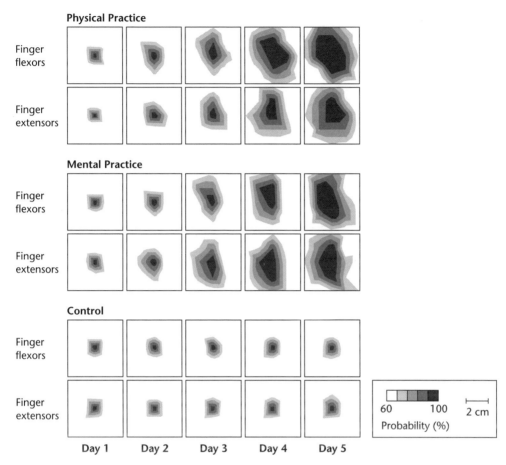

Figure 6 *Experiment 2*: representative examples of the cortical motor output maps for the long finger flexor and extensor muscles on *days 1–5* in a subject from each group. Each map is based on 25 measured points.

of function (Cohen et al., 1991b, 1993; Pascual-Leone et al., 1992). These findings confirm in humans the growing body of evidence suggesting the flexible nature of connections in the nervous system of adult animals (Kaas 1991).

The nervous system of animals may also undergo changes according to the patterns of use, thereby providing a substrate for the acquisition of new skills (Jenkins et al., 1990; Merzenich et al., 1990). The sensorimotor representation of the preferred hand in monkeys is more elaborate than that of the nonpreferred hand (Nudo et al., 1992), and training can result in distortions of body surface and movement representations that lead to behavioral gains (Jenkins et al., 1990). Motor cortical representation of a body part expands after selectively increased activity (Humphrey et al., 1990; Sanes et al., 1992), and differential stimulation of a restricted skin surface in a finger pad of adult monkeys leads to a reorganization of its somatosensory cortical representation, especially when stimulation has a functional significance (Recanzone et al., 1992a–d). In humans, a recent positron emission tomography study (Seitz et al., 1990) found that

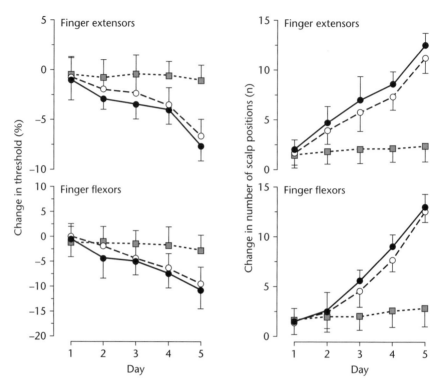

Figure 7 *Experiment 2*: change in motor threshold, expressed as a percentage of the baseline threshold, and in number of scalp positions from which MEPs could be produced in the long finger flexor and extensor muscles with a probability of ≥60 per cent in all subjects (mean ± SD) over the course of 5 days. Filled circles, physical practice group; open circles, mental practice group; stippled squares, control group.

learning of a complicated sequence of voluntary finger movements is associated with increases in regional cerebral blood flow (rCBF) in the cerebellum and that acquisition of the motor skill results in an increase of rCBF in the striatum. Relative increases in rCBF have been shown to occur in the primary motor area, the supplementary motor area, and the thalamus as subjects learned a pursuit rotor task (Grafton et al., 1992). Finally, changes in slow cortical negative DC potentials during the acquisition of a complex finger motor task (Niemann et al., 1991) also suggest a dynamic modulation of the cortical representation of movement control during skill learning.

In the present study we found that acquisition of the motor skills needed for the correct performance of a five-finger piano exercise is associated with modulation of the cortical motor outputs to the muscles involved in the task. The cortical sensorimotor representation of a specific body part, as demonstrated, for example, by TMS mapping, may depend on the momentary level of excitability of the intracortical network that targets it. Extensive intracortical axonal collaterals provide inputs to many different movement representations of a given body part, and their pattern of recruitment may determine the execution of complex movements (Huntley and Jones 1991). In addition, neuronal networks targeting different body parts overlap widely and even share in part common neuronal elements (Schieber 1992). The neuronal elements in such networks may maintain a flexible balance based on demand and competition by their targets. Removal of a target, as in amputation or peripheral deafferentation, may result in the 'takeover' of neuronal elements, formerly activated primarily as part of the network targeting the removed target, by neighboring networks targeting neighboring body parts. This would explain the reorganization of the motor outputs targeting muscles proximal to the stump of an amputated limb (Cohen et al., 1991a) or to an ischemic sensorimotor block (Brasil-Neto et al., 1992, 1993). Conversely, increased use and enhanced sensory feedback of a body part, especially if coupled with functional gain for the subject, may lead to a shift of the balance of intracortical networks toward that body part. Cortical networks underlying coordinated finger movements show a movement gradient across digits from the most prominently activated digit, which may depend on corticocortical or sub-corticocortical projections (Amassian et al., 1989). Learning and practice may modulate the cortical outputs by strengthening such a gradient.

Modulation of motor cortical outputs may result from the establishment or unmasking of neuronal connections. The rapid time course of the motor output modulation, by which a certain region of motor cortex can increase its influence on a motoneuron pool, suggests the unmasking of existing neuronal connections, which may be due to decreased inhibition or increased synaptic efficacy (long-term potentiation) (Asanuma and Keller 1991; Iriki et al., 1989; Jacobs and Donoghue 1991). Such flexible modulation may represent a first stage in learning and could lead to structural changes in the intracortical and subcortical networks as the skill becomes overlearned and automatic. For example, Greenough et al. (Greenough 1984; Greenough et al., 1985) have shown that motor training is associated with changes in the dendritic branching patterns of motor and sensory cortical cells involved in the performance of the task. Sprouting may account for plastic changes in such situations, as likely occurred in monkeys deafferented for 10 years (Pons et al., 1991), and represents the correlate of long-standing 'memories.'

Learning-associated modulation of motor cortical outputs may result from changes in synaptic efficacy in the motor cortex itself (Jacobs and Donoghue 1991). However, our results do not allow ruling out that the observed plastic changes are driven by changes in the activity of other cortical areas or subcortical structures, for example, the premotor cortex or the cerebellum. Discharge patterns of Purkinje cells change during motor learning (Gilbert and Thach 1977; Ojakangas and Ebner 1992), which could lead to changes in cortical excitability via cerebellothalamocortical projections. A large proportion of cells in the premotor cortex in the monkey show a learning-dependent change in activity during the acquisition of visuomotor associations (Mitz et al., 1991), which could modulate primary motor cortex activity via cortico-cortical projections. Even a shift in the segmental excitability of appropriate spinal levels could account for the observed changes in the motor outputs. For example, an excitatory input to α-motoneurons from suprasegmental levels or increased fusiform drive could bring the motoneurons close to firing level without overtly causing background EMG. Further studies are needed to define the level of the observed plasticity.

The changes in cortical motor outputs that we observed during TMS do not necessarily reflect the cortical activation pattern evoked during task performance, because TMS was applied while the subject was at rest, not performing the trained task.

Therefore they must indicate a longer-lasting change possibly due to long-term synaptic potentiation (Asanuma and Keller 1991; Iriki et al., 1989; Jacobs and Donoghue 1991). We show that the 'momentary level of excitability,' a fixed time after performance of the task (20 min to ~3 h), rises progressively over the course of 5 days for the cortical outputs to muscles involved in the task as the subject's performance improves. Further practice may eventually lead to new changes in the cortical motor outputs as the task becomes overlearned and correct performance eventually may become 'automatic' (Pascual-Leone et al., 1994). An important issue raised by our findings is the apparent lack of a plateau in the modulation of cortical outputs during learning. We believe that this apparent lack of plateau is likely an artifact of the duration of our study design. Our assumption would be that if we would continue with the training of the task used in the present study for longer than a week, there would be a plateau of the cortical output changes and even possibly a return of cortical thresholds to baseline as the skill becomes overlearned.

Effect of manual and mental practice

Mental practice is the imagined rehearsal of a motor act with the specific intent of learning or improving it, without overt movement output. Mental practice can be viewed as a virtual simulation of behavior by which the subject develops and 'internally' rehearses a cognitive representation of the motor act. When confronted with a new motor task, the subject must develop a cognitive representation of it and initiate a centrally guided response, which secondarily can be improved by the use of sensorimotor feedback. Mental practice may accelerate the acquisition of a new motor skill by providing a well-suited cognitive model of the demanded motor act in advance of any physical practice (McBride and Rothstein 1979; Mendoza and Wichman 1978; White et al., 1979). Mental practice has found wide acceptance in the training of athletes (Denis 1985; Suinn 1984), and several famous instrumental musicians have used mental practice in the learning and rehearsal of new compositions (Schönberg 1987, 1988).

Studies of rCBF suggest that the prefrontal and supplementary motor areas, basal ganglia, and cerebellum are part of the network involved in the mental simulation of motor acts (Decety and Ingvar 1990; Ingvar and Philipson 1977; Roland et al., 1980, 1982, 1987; Roland and Friberg 1985). Therefore mental simulation of movements activates some of the same central neural structures required for the performance of the actual movements. In doing so, mental practice alone seems to be sufficient to promote the modulation of neural circuits involved in the early stages of motor skill learning. This modulation not only results in marked performance improvement but also seems to place the subjects at an advantage for further skill learning with minimal physical practice. The combination of mental and physical practice leads to greater performance improvement than physical practice alone (McBride and Rothstein 1979; White et al., 1979), a phenomenon for which our findings provide a physiological explanation. Mental imaging of movements recreates the effects of physical practice on the modulation of the central motor system and may, therefore, be an important adjunct not only for the learning of new motor skills but also for the maintenance of motor skills in temporarily immobilized patients and in the rehabilitation of patients with neurological disorders.

References

Amassian, V.E., Cracco, R.Q. and Maccabee, P.J. Focal stimulation of the human cerebral cortex with magnetic coil: a comparison with electrical stimulation. *Electroencephalogr. Clin. Neurophysiol.* 74: 401–416, 1989.

Aou, S.A., Woody, C.D. and Birt, D. Increases in excitability of neurons of the motor cortex of cats after rapid acquisition of eye blink conditioning. *J. Neurophysiol.* 12: 560–569, 1992.

Asanuma, H. and Keller, A. Neuronal mechanisms of motor learning in mammals. *Neuroreport* 2: 217–24, 1991.

Brasil-Neto, J.P., Cohen, L.G., Pascual-Leone, A., Jabir, F.K., Wall, R.T. and Hallett, M. Rapid reversible reorganization in human motor system following transient deafferentation. *Neurology* 42: 1302–1306, 1992.

Brasil-Neto, J.P., Valls-Solé, J., Pascual-Leone, A., Cammarota, A., Amassian, V.E., Cracco, R., Maccabee, P., Cracco, J., Hallett, M. and Cohen, L.G. Rapid modulation of human cortical motor outputs following ischaemic nerve block. *Brain* 116: 511–525, 1993.

Cohen, L.G., Bandinelli, S., Findlay, T.W. and Hallett, M. Motor reorganization after upper limb amputation in man. *Brain* 114: 615–627, 1991a.

Cohen, L.G., Brasil-Neto, J.P., Pascual-Leone, A. and Hallett, M. Plasticity of cortical motor output organization following deafferentation, cerebral lesions, and skill acquisition. *Adv. Neurol.* 63: 187–200, 1993.

Cohen, L.G., Roth, B.J., Nilsson, J., Dang, N., Bandinelli, S., Panizza, M., Friauf, W. and Hallett, M. Effects of coil design on delivery of focal magnetic stimulation. Technical considerations. *Electroencephalogr. Clin. Neurophysiol.* 75: 350–357, 1990.

Cohen, L.G., Roth, B.J., Wassermann, E.M., Topka, H., Fuhr, P., Schultz, J. and Hallett, M. Magnetic stimulation of the human cerebral cortex, an indicator of reorganization in motor pathways in certain pathological conditions. *J. Clin. Neurophysiol.* 8: 56–65, 1991b.

Decety, J. and Ingvar, D.H. Brain structures participating in mental simulation of motor behavior: a neuropsychological interpretation. *Acta Psychol.* 73: 13–34, 1990.

Denis, M. Visual imagery and the use of mental practice in the development of motor skills. *Can. J. Appl. Sport Sci.* 10: 4S–16S, 1985.

Gilbert, P.F.C. and Thach, W. T. Purkinje cell activity during motor learning. *Brain Res.* 128: 309–328, 1977.

Grafton, S.T., Mazziotta, J.C., Presty, S., Friston, K.J., Frackowiak, R.S.J. and Phleps, M.E. Functional anatomy of human procedural learning determined with regional cerebral blood flow and PET. *J. Neurosci.* 12: 2542–2548, 1992.

Greenough, W.T. Structural correlates of information storage in the mammalian brain: a review and hypothesis. *Trends Neurosci.* 7: 229–233, 1984.

Greenough, W.T., Larson, J.R. and Withers, G.S. Effects of unilateral and bilateral training in a reaching task on dendritic branching of neurons in the rat motor-sensory forelimb cortex. *Behav. Neural Biol.* 44: 301–314, 1985.

Humphrey, D.R., Oiu, X.O., Clavel, P. and O'Donoghue, D.L. Changes in forelimb motor representation in rodent cortex induced by passive movements. *Soc. Neurosci. Abstr.* 16: 422, 1990.

Huntley, G.W. and Jones, E.G. Relationship of intrinsic connections to forelimb movement representations in monkey cortex: a correlative anatomic and physiological study. *J. Neurophysiol.* 66: 390–413, 1991.

Ingvar, D.H. and Philipson, L. Distribution of the cerebral blood flow in the dominant hemisphere during motor ideation and motor performance. *Ann. Neurol.* 2: 230–237, 1977.

Iriki, A., Pavlides, C., Keller, A. and Asanuma, H. Long-term potentiation of motor cortex. *Science Wash. DC* 245: 1385–1387, 1989.

Jacobs, K.M. and Donoghue, J.P. Reshaping the cortical motor map by unmasking latent intracortical connections. *Science Wash. DC* 251: 944–947, 1991.

Jenkins, W.M., Merzenich, M.M. and Recanzone, G. Neocortical representational dynamics in adult primates: implications for neuropsychology. *Neuropsychologia* 28: 573–584, 1990.

Kaas, J.H. Plasticity of sensory and motor maps in adult mammals. *Annu. Rev. Neurosci.* 14: 137–167, 1991.

Levy, W.J., Amassian, V.E., Schimd, U.D. and Jungreis, C. Mapping of motor cortex gyral sites non-invasively by transcranial magnetic stimulation in normal subjects and patients. In: *Magnetic Motor Stimulation: Basic Principles and Clinical Experience,* edited by W.J. Levy, R.Q. Cracco, A.T. Barker and J. Rothwell. Amsterdam: Elsevier, 1991, pp. 51–75.

Maccabee, P.J., Amassian, V.E., Eberle, L. and Cracco, R.Q. Magnetic coil stimulation of straight and bent amphibian and mammalian peripheral nerve in vitro: locus of excitation. *J. Physiol. Lond.* 460: 201–219, 1993.

Maccabee, P.J., Eberle, L., Amassian, V.E., Cracco, R.Q., Rudell, A.P. and Jayachandra, M. Spatial distribution of the electric field induced in volume by a round and figure '8' magnetic coils: relevance to activation of sensory nerve fibers. *Electroencephalogr. Clin. Neurophysiol.* 76: 131–141, 1990.

McBride, E.R. and Rothstein, A.L. Mental and physical practice and the learning and retention of open and closed skills. *Percept. Mot. Skills* 49: 359–365, 1979.

Mendoza, D.W. and Wichman, H. 'Inner' darts: effects of mental practice on performance of dart throwing. *Percept. Mot. Skills* 47: 1195–1199, 1978.

Merzenich, M.M., Recanzone, G.H., Jenkins, W.M. and Grajski, K.A. Adaptive mechanisms in cortical networks underlying cortical contributions to learning and nondeclarative memory. *Cold Spring Harbor Symp. Quant. Biol.* 55: 873–887, 1990.

Mitz, A.R., Godschalk, M. and Wise, S.P. Learning-dependent neuronal activity in the premotor cortex: activity during the acquisition of conditional motor associations. *J. Neurosci.* 11: 1855–1872, 1991.

Niemann, J., Winker, T., Gerling, J., Landwehrmeyer, B. and Jung, R. Changes in slow cortical negative DC-potentials during the acquisition of a complex finger motor task. *Exp. Brain Res.* 85: 417–422, 1991.

Nudo, R.J., Jenkins, W.M., Merzenich, M.M., Prejean, T. and Grenda, R. Neurophysiological correlates of hand preference in primary motor cortex of adult squirrel monkeys. *J. Neurosci.* 12: 2918–2947, 1992.

Ojakangas, C.L. and Ebner, T.J. Purkinje cell complex and simple spike changes during a voluntary arm movement learning task in the monkey. *J. Neurophysiol.* 68: 2222–2236, 1992.

Oldfield, R.C. The assessment and analysis of handedness: the Edinburgh inventory. *Neuropsychologia* 9: 97–113, 1971.

Pascual-Leone, A., Cammarota, A., Wassermann, E.M., Cohen, L.G. and Hallett, M. Modulation of motor cortical outputs to the reading hand of Braille readers. *Ann. Neurol.* 34: 33–37, 1993.

Pascual-Leone, A., Cohen, L.G. and Hallett, M. Noninvasive evaluation of plastic changes in human motor system. *Trends Neurosci.* 15: 13–15, 1992.

Pascual-Leone, A., Grafman, J. and Hallett, M. Modulation of cortical motor output maps during the development of implicit and explicit knowledge. *Science Wash. DC* 263: 1287–1289, 1994.

Pascual-Leone, A. and Torres, F. Plasticity of the sensorimotor cortex representation of the reading finger in Braille readers. *Brain* 116: 39–52, 1993.

Pons, T.P., Garraghty, P.E., Ommaya, A.K., Kass, J.H., Taub, E. and Mishkin, M. Massive cortical reorganization after sensory deafferentation in adult macaques. *Science Wash. DC* 252: 1857–1860, 1991.

Recanzone, G.H., Jenkins, W.M., Hradek, G.T. and Merzenich, M.M. Progressive improvement in discriminative abilities in adult owl monkeys performing a tactile frequency discrimination task. *J. Neurophysiol.* 67: 1015–1030, 1992a.

Recanzone, G.H., Merzenich, M.M. and Jenkins, W.M. Frequency discrimination training engaging a restricted skin surface results in an emergence of a cutaneous response zone in cortical area 3a. *J. Neurophysiol.* 67: 1057–1070, 1992b.

Recanzone, G.H., Merzenich, M.M., Jenkins, W.M., Grajski, K.A. and Dinse, H.R. Topographic reorganization of the hand representation in cortical area 3b owl monkeys trained in a frequency-discrimination task. *J. Neurophysiol.* 67: 1031–1056, 1992c.

Recanzone, G.H., Merzenich, M.M. and Schreiner, C.E. Changes in the distributed temporal response properties of SI cortical neurons reflect improvements in performance on a temporally based tactile discrimination task. *J. Neurophysiol.* 67: 1071–1091, 1992d.

Roland, P.E., Ericksson, L., Stone-Elander, S. and Widen, L. Does mental activity change the oxidative metabolism of the brain? *J. Neurosci.* 7: 2373–2389, 1987.

Roland, P.E. and Friberg, L. Localization of cortical areas activated by thinking. *J. Neurophysiol.* 53: 1219–1243, 1985.

Roland, P.E., Larsen, B., Lassen, N.A. and Skinhoj, E. Supplementary motor area and other cortical areas in organization of voluntary movements in man. *J. Neurophysiol.* 43: 118–136, 1980.

Roland, P.E., Meyer, E., Shibasaki, T., Yamamoto, Y.L. and Thompson, C.J. Regional cerebral blood flow changes in cortex and ganglia during voluntary movements in normal human volunteers. *J. Neurophysiol.* 48: 467–478, 1982.

Roth, B.J., Cohen, L.G. and Hallett, M. The electric field induced during transcranial magnetic stimulation. *Electroencephalogr. Clin. Neurophysiol. Suppl.* 43: 268–278, 1991a.

Roth, B.J., Saypol, J.M., Hallett, M. and Cohen, L.G. A theoretical calculation of the electric field induced in the cortex during magnetic stimulation. *Electroencephalogr. Clin. Neurophysiol.* 81: 47–56, 1991b.

Sanes, J.N., Wang, J. and Donoghue, J.P. Immediate and delayed changes of rat motor cortical output representation with new forelimb configurations. *Cereb. Cortex* 2: 141–152, 1992.

Schieber, M.H. Widely distributed neuron activity in primary motor cortex area during individuated finger movements. *Soc. Neurosci. Abstr.* 18: 504, 1992.

Schonberg, H. *Great Pianists*. St. Louis, MO: Fireside Books, 1987.

Schonberg, H. *The Virtuosi*. New York: Vintage-Random House, 1988.

Seitz, R.J., Roland, E., Bohm, C., Greitz, T. and Stone-Elander, S. Motor learning in man: a positron emission tomographic study. *Neuroreport* 1: 57–60, 1990.

Suinn, R.M. Imagery and sport. In: *Imagery and Sport*, edited by W.F. Straub and J.M. Williams. Lansing, NY: Sport Science Associates, 1984.

Tofts, P.S. The distribution of induced currents in magnetic stimulation of the nervous system. *Phys. Med. Biol.* 35: 1119–1128, 1990.

Wassermann, E.M., McShane, L.M., Hallett, M. and Cohen, L.G. Noninvasive mapping of muscle representations in human motor cortex. *Electroencephalogr. Clin. Neurophysiol.* 85: 1–12, 1991.

Wassermann, E.M., Wang, B., Toro, C., Zeffiro, T., Valls-Solé, J., Pascual-Leone, A. and Hallett, M. Projecting transcranial magnetic stimulation (TMS) maps into brain MRI. *Soc. Neurosci. Abstr.* 18: 939, 1992.

White, C.A., Ashton, R. and Lewis, S. Learning a complex skill: effect of mental practice, physical practice and imagery ability. *Int. J. Sports Psychol.* 10: 71–78, 1979.

Appendix 2 – Chapter 3

Research report

Premotor cortex and the recognition of motor actions

Rizzolatti, G., Fadiga, L., Gallese, V. and Fogassi, L. (1996)
Cognitive Brain Research, 3(2): 131–41.

Abstract

In area F5 of the monkey premotor cortex there are neurons that discharge both when the monkey performs an action and when he observes a similar action made by another monkey or by the experimenter. We report here some of the properties of these 'mirror' neurons and we propose that their activity 'represents' the observed action. We posit, then, that this motor representation is at the basis of the under-standing of motor events. Finally, on the basis of some recent data showing that, in man, the observation of motor actions activate the posterior part of inferior frontal gyrus, we suggest that the development of the lateral verbal communication system in man derives from a more ancient communication system based on recognition of hand and face gestures.

Keywords: Premotor cortex; Mirror neuron; Gesture recognition; Broca's area; Movement representation

1. Introduction

An important discovery of the last years was that the monkey agranular frontal cortex is functionally subdivided into several different areas [10,11,19,24,27,28,33–35,37,38,54]. Among them one – area F5 – is particularly interesting for its complex properties and for its possible homology with Broca's area of human brain [2,15,42].

F5 is located in the ventro-rostral part of area 6, just caudal to the lower arm of the arcuate sulcus. Stimulation and recording experiments showed that this area is related to hand and mouth movements [20,24,52,55]. F5 has a rough somatotopic organization. Hand movements are represented mostly in its dorsal part, while mouth movements tend to be represented ventrally.

While little is known about the properties of F5 neurons related to mouth move-ments, the properties of those controlling hand movements were extensively studied. Hand-movement F5 neurons have both motor and sensory properties. As far as the motor properties are concerned, two are their main characteristics. Firstly, most neurons discharge selectively during particular goal-related hand movements such as grasping, holding, manipulating. Secondly, many of them are specific for particular types of hand prehension, e.g. precision grip, finger prehension, whole hand prehension. For the sensory properties, the most interesting aspect is that a considerable part of F5 neurons fire at the presentation of 3D objects, in the absence of any overt movement. In many cases the discharge occurs only if there is a match between the object size and the type of grip coded by the neuron [22,52].

F5 receives a strong input from the inferior parietal lobule [6,31,47] and, in particular, from area AIP [16,22,32], an area located in the lateral bank of the inferior parietal sulcus rostral to the oculomotor area LIP. As in the case of F5, a large number of neurons in AIP are related to hand movements, the large majority preferring specific types of hand grip [57,58]. About 40 per cent of AIP neurons discharge during the appropriate hand movement both in darkness or in the light (motor dominant neurons). The remaining neurons discharge stronger (visual and motor neurons) or exclusively (visual dominant neurons) in the light. A part of neurons of these last classes become active when the monkey fixates an appropriate object remaining still and without being required to make a movement toward it.

Taken together, these data indicate that AIP and F5 form a cortical circuit which transforms visual information on the intrinsic properties of the objects into hand movements that allow the animal to interact appropriately with the objects. Motor information is then transferred to F1, to which F5 is directly connected, as well as to various subcortical centers for movement execution [22].

Recently we discovered that a particular subset of F5 neurons, which from the motor point of view are undistinguishable from the rest of the population, discharge when the monkey observes meaningful hand movements made by the experimenter ('mirror neurons') [9]. The effective experimenter's movements included, among others, placing or taking away objects from a table, grasping food from another experimenter, manipulating objects. There was always a link between the effective observed movement and the effective executed movement.

These data suggest that area F5 is endowed with an observation/execution matching system. When the monkey observes a motor action that belongs (or resembles) its movement repertoire, this action is automatically retrieved. The retrieved action is not necessarily executed. It is only represented in the motor system. We speculated that this observation/execution mechanism plays a role in understanding the meaning of motor events [9,22].

The main aim of the present article is to discuss this proposal, taking into consideration some recent data showing that an observation/execution matching system does exists in man [13] and that the cortical region involved in this matching is a part of the region usually referred to as Broca's area [53]. Since this article means to be essentially a theoretical article, in the Results section we will present only a description of the most important features of 'mirror' neurons and will show some examples of them. A detailed description of these neurons and all the control experiments (e.g. EMG recordings, recordings from F1 neurons) that we performed in order to exclude that 'mirror' effect could be due to monkey's movements or other spurious factors will be presented elsewhere.

2.   **Materials and methods**

2.1.   **Recording**

Single neurons were recorded from two unanesthetized, behaving monkeys (*Macaca nemestrina*). All experimental protocols were approved by the Veterinarian Animal Care and Use Committee of the University of Parma and complied with the European law on the humane care and use of laboratory animals.

The surgical procedures for neuron recordings were the same as previously described [17,54]. The head implant included a head holder and a chamber for single-unit recordings. Neurons were recorded using tungsten micro-electrodes inserted through the dura which was left intact. Neuronal activity was amplified and monitored on an oscilloscope. Individual action potentials were isolated with a time-amplitude voltage discriminator. The output signal from the voltage discriminator was monitored and fed to a PC for analysis.

2.2.   **'Clinical' testing and behavioral paradigm**

All neurons were first informally tested by showing the monkey objects of different size and shape, and by letting him grasp them (for details see [17,52]). Every time a neuron became active during the monkey's hand movements, its properties were studied in a behaviorally controlled situation. A testing box was placed in front of the monkey. The box front door was formed by a one-way mirror. The room illumination was such that the monkey could not see inside the box during intertrial periods. Geometric solids of different size and shape were placed inside the box. The monkey started each trial by pressing a switch. Switch lit the box and made the object visible. After a delay of 1.2–1.5 s, the box front door opened, thus allowing the monkey to reach for and grasp the object. The animal was rewarded with a piece of food located in a well under the object. Arm and hand movements were recorded using a computerized movement recording system (ELITE System, see [14]). This system consists of two infrared TV-cameras and a processor which elaborates the video images in real time and reconstructs the 3D position of infrared reflecting markers. The markers used for reconstructing the monkey's hand and arm movements were placed on the first phalanges of the thumb and the index finger and on the radial apophysis.

2.3.   **Testing of 'mirror' properties**

'Mirror' properties were tested by performing a series of motor actions in front of the monkey. These actions were related to food grasping (e.g. presenting the food to the monkey, putting it on a surface, grasping it, giving it to a second experimenter or taking it away from him), to manipulation of food or other objects (e.g. breaking, tearing, folding), or were intransitive gestures (non-object related) with or without 'emotional' content (e.g. threatening gestures, lifting the arms, waving the hand, etc.).

In order to verify whether the recorded neuron coded specifically hand–object interactions, the following actions were also performed: movements of the hand mimicking grasping in the absence of the object; prehension movements of food or other objects performed with tools (e.g. forceps, pincers); simultaneous combined movements of the food and hand, spatially separated one from the other. All experimenter's actions were repeated on the right and on the left of the monkey at various distances (50 cm, 1 m and 2 m).

The animal's behavior and the experimenters' actions during testing of complex visual properties were recorded on one track of a videotape. The neural activity was simultaneously recorded on a second track, in order to correlate the monkey's behavior or the experimenters' actions to the neuron's discharge. When possible, response histograms were also constructed using a contact detecting circuit for aligning behavioral events and neuron's discharge.

2.4. Histological identification

After the last experiment the animal was anesthetized with ketamine (15 mg/kg, i.m.) and, after an additional dose of sodium thiopental (30–40 mg, i.v.), perfused through the left ventricle with warm buffered saline followed by fixative (for details, see [33]). The animal was then placed in the stereotaxic apparatus, the dura was removed, and the stereotaxic coordinates of the arcuate and central sulci were assessed. The brain was blocked coronally on a stereotaxic frame, removed from the skull, photographed, and then frozen and cut coronally (each section: 60 μm). Alternate sections were stained with the Nissl method and reacted for cytochrome oxidase histochemistry. The locations of the penetrations were reconstructed and related to the various cytochrome oxidase areas of the frontal agranular cortex [33].

3. Results

Figure 1 shows a lateral view of the monkey brain. 'Mirror neurons' were recorded from the dorsal convexity of the cortex (shadowed area) and the adjacent posterior bank of the arcuate sulcus. Both these cortices are part of area F5. Mirror neurons represented, approximately, 20 per cent of the recorded neurons ($n = 300$).

With the term 'mirror neurons' we indicated those neurons that became active when the monkey observed meaningful hand actions performed by the experimenter. The simple presentation of objects, even when held by hand, did not evoke the neuron discharge. The majority of mirror neurons (about 60 per cent) were selective for one type of action (e.g. grasping). Some were highly specific, selectively firing during the observation of a particular type of hand configuration used to grasp or manipulate an object (e.g. precision grip, but not whole hand prehension). The remaining neurons were activated by the observation of two or more hand actions. The actions most represented were: grasp, put object on a surface in front of the monkey, manipulate.

A typical example of a mirror neuron is presented in Figure 2. In Figure 2A (left part) the monkey observes the experimenter grasping a small piece of food placed on a tray. The tray is then moved towards the monkey and the monkey grasps the food (right part). The neuron discharges when the experimenter grasps the food, stops firing when the food is moved towards the monkey, and discharges again when the monkey

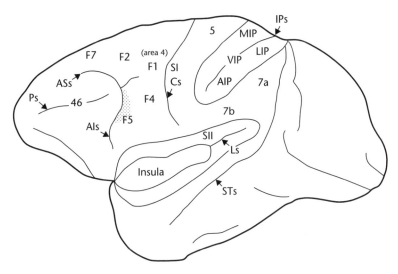

Figure 1 Lateral view of the monkey brain. The shaded area shows the anatomical localization of the recorded neurons. Frontal agranular cortical areas are classified according to Matelli et al. [33]. Abbreviations: AIP, anterior intraparietal area; AIs, inferior arcuate sulcus; ASs, superior arcuate sulcus; Cs, central sulcus; IPs, intraparietal sulcus; LIP, lateral intraparietal area; Ls, lateral sulcus; MIP, medial intraparietal area; Ps, principal sulcus; SI, primary somatosensory area; SII, secondary somatosensory area; STs, superior temporal sulcus; VIP, ventral intraparietal area. Note that IPs and Ls have been opened to show hidden areas.

grasps the food. In Figure 2B the experimenter grasps the food using a tool, then, as in Figure 2A, gives the food to the monkey. In this case there is no response during action observation. The neuron fires only during monkey's grasping.

The discharge pattern illustrated in Figure 2A is typical of mirror neurons. Note that there was no response when food was moved toward the monkey and became therefore available to him. This absence of response just before the actual movement allows one to rule out motor preparation as a possible explanation for the neuron's activation during grasping observation.

The interaction between hand and object (Figure 2A) was a fundamental requisite for neuron activation. Hand movements performed without an object did not activate the neurons. This was usually true also when food was grasped with a tool (Figure 2B). In this last situation only few neurons became active and, in most cases, much less than during hand movements. Covering the object with a container (e.g. a beaker), with a cardboard, or removing it from the monkey's view together with the surface on which it was located did not activate mirror neurons.

The great majority of mirror neurons (79 per cent) had also motor properties. The possibility that the discharges associated with active movements were due to the monkey's vision of his own hand was controlled by recording neuron activity during grasping made in darkness. All neurons were found to be active in this condition. Figure 2C illustrates this finding.

(A)

(B)

(C)

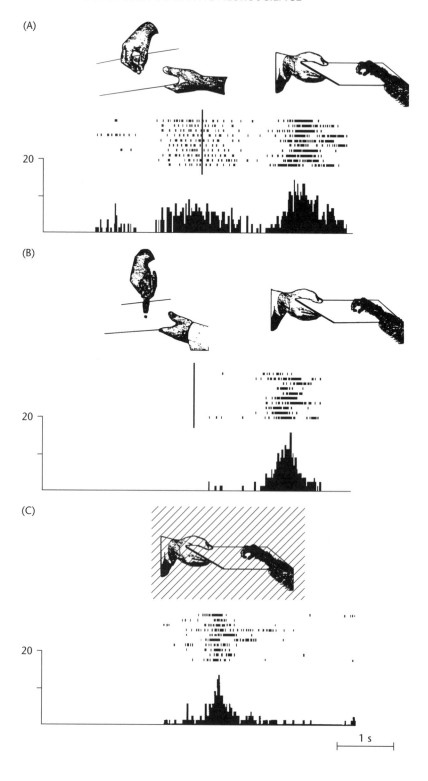

1 s

A comparison carried out in each mirror neuron between the effective visual stimuli and the effective active movements, showed the presence of different degrees of congruence. A very high degree of congruence was found in those neurons that, being highly specific in their motor properties, were also highly specific in their visual properties. In these neurons the action coded in motor terms coincided with the action that, when seen, triggered the neuron.

The activity of a highly congruent mirror neuron is illustrated in Figure 3. This neuron discharged when the experimenter rotated his hands in opposite directions around a small piece of food, as if for breaking it (Figure 3A). Neither the observation of grasping movements, nor active grasping (Figure 3C) triggered the neuron. When the monkey made wrist rotations in order to take away the food from the experimenter's hand, a brisk response appeared (Figure 3B).

Another example of a congruent neuron is illustrated in Figure 4. Also in this case the only visual stimulus capable to activate the neuron was the observation of an action similar to that coded by the neuron. Figure 4A shows that the observation of the experimenter placing a piece of food on a tray did not modify the discharge rate of the neuron. The discharge, however, was strongly inhibited during the observation of the experimenter grasping the same piece of food (Figure 4B). The neuron's discharge was also strongly inhibited when the monkey grasped the food (Figure 4C).

A broader type of congruence between the observed and the executed action was found in those neurons which could be activated by several visually related observed actions (such as different types of prehension or different actions such as placing and grasping) beside the one corresponding to the monkey's effective movement. Only few neurons did not show any relation between the effective observed and executed actions.

The specificity of most mirror neurons and the congruence observed in many of them between the observed and executed effective actions, renders very unlikely that their activation during gesture observation was due to monkey–experimenter interactions related to unspecific factors such as food expectancy, motor preparation for food retrieval or reward. In order, however, to control for these possibilities, we tested a group of mirror neurons using a second monkey as a performer of the actions. During this testing the recorded monkey had his hands restrained and did not receive food.

Figure 2 (*opposite*) Visual and motor responses of a mirror neuron. The behavioral situations are schematically represented in the upper part of each panel. In the lower part are shown a series of consecutive rasters and the relative peristimulus response histograms. A, the experimenter grasps a piece of food with his hand and moves it towards the monkey who, at the end of the trial, grasps it. The neuron discharges during grasping observation, ceases to fire when the food is moved and discharges again when the monkey grasps it. B, the experimenter grasps the food with a tool. Subsequent sequence of events as in A. The neuron response during action observation is absent. C, the monkey grasps food in the darkness. In A and B the rasters are aligned with the moment in which the food is grasped by the experimenter (vertical line across the rasters). In C the alignment is with the approximate beginning of the grasping movement. Histogram bin width: 20 ms. Ordinates, spikes/bin; abscissae, time.

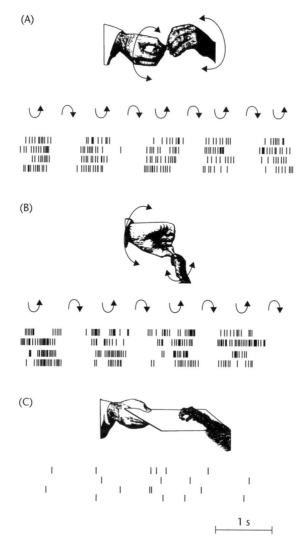

Figure 3 Example of a highly congruent mirror neuron. A, the monkey observes the experimenter who rotates his hands around a raisin in opposite directions alternating clockwise and counterclockwise movements. The response is present only in one rotation direction. B, the experimenter rotates a piece of food held by the monkey who opposes the experimenter movement making a wrist rotation movement in the opposite direction. C, monkey grasps food using a precision grip. Four continuous recordings are shown in each panel. Small arrows above the records indicate the direction of rotations.

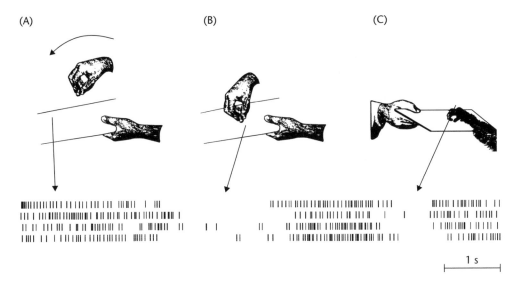

Figure 4 Example of another highly congruent mirror neuron. A, the experimenter places a raisin on a tray. B, the experimenter grasps the same raisin. C, the monkey grasps the raisin. A response inhibition of the spontaneous discharge is present during active grasping and grasping observation. The two responses are indicated by the second and the third arrow. No changes in the spontaneous activity is present when the monkey observes the experimenter placing the food on the tray (first arrow). Four continuous recordings are shown.

One of these experiments is illustrated in Figure 5. The neuron was activated both when the recorded monkey observed grasping movements made by the second monkey (Figure 5A) or made by the experimenter (Figure 5B). There was also a strong response associated with grasping movements executed by the recorded monkey (Figure 5C).

4. **Discussion**

4.1. Neurophysiological findings

Neurons that are selectively activated by complex biologically meaningful visual stimuli have been observed in many high-order cortical areas [5,8,18,41,44,45,49] and in the amygdala [4,26]. These neurons respond to the sight of hands, faces and particular types of body movements. Among them there are neurons, located in the depth of the superior temporal sulcus, that are specifically responsive to hand–object interactions [44,46].

Mirror neurons of area F5 share with these 'complex' neurons the property of being responsive to meaningful stimuli. They differ, however, from these neurons in that they discharge also during movements performed by the observer that mimic the

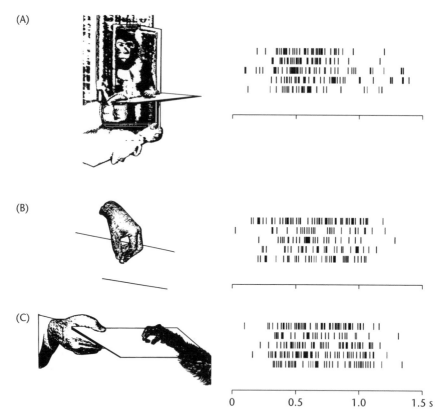

Figure 5 Activation of a mirror neuron during the observation of grasping movements performed by a monkey seated in front of the recorded monkey (A), by the experimenter (B) and during the execution of grasping performed by the recorded monkey (C). Each panel illustrates five records of 1.5 s. The spontaneous activity was virtually absent. The neuron discharge was triggered either by the observation or execution of grasping movements.

actions whose observation activate them. Neurons with mirror properties have been described up to now only in F5. It is likely, however, that they are not unique to this area, but do exist in other frontal and parietal cortical areas that control the organization of goal directed movements.

What may the functional role of mirror neurons be? Do they exist also in man? And if this is so, where can they be located? In the following discussion we will try to answer these questions.

4.2. Possible functional role of mirror neurons

An explanation of mirror neurons that comes naturally to mind is that they are related to motor preparation. When the monkey observes an action, he starts automatically to prepare the same action. In this way he becomes able to perform it fast, thus prevailing on possible competitors. If this explanation is accepted, mirror neurons would be nothing else but a particular type of 'set-related neurons' (see [59,60]). These are a rather common type of premotor neurons that start to fire in advance of movement execution, when its target is prespecified. The 'preparation' explanation is unsatisfactory for two reasons. First, the discharge of mirror neurons caused by the observation of a movement is not followed by the movement that, supposedly, was prepared. The monkey looking at an another monkey that grasps food does not move subsequently his fingers. Secondly, and most importantly, mirror neurons cease firing when the food is moved toward the animal and becomes available to him. If the firing of mirror neurons were related to motor preparation, the neuron activity should have increased and not decreased in the phase that precedes movement execution.

A more sophisticated interpretation of mirror neurons was given by Jeannerod [21]. In a recent review article on motor imagery he made the example of a pupil learning how to play a musical instrument. The pupil is completely still, watching the teacher who demonstrates an action that he must imitate and reproduce later. Although the pupil is immobile, he must form an image in his brain of the teacher's action. Jeannerod's view is that the neurons responsible for the motor image formation are the same the pupil will later activate during planning and preparation of the action. According to him mirror neurons are neurons that internally 'represent' an action.

The explanation we favor is similar to that proposed by Jeannerod. We also think that mirror neurons are neurons that 'represent' internally actions. However, whereas the emphasis given by Jeannerod is on learning, our view is that mirror neurons play a role in the understanding of motor events [9].

By the term 'understanding motor events' we do not imply self-conciousness (see [51]). With this term we indicate only the capacity of an individual to recognize the presence of another individual performing an action, to differentiate the observed action from other actions, and to use this information in order to act appropriately. Some of the mechanisms mediating operations of this type are linked to emotion and depend on the integrity of limbic structures (see [3]). Lesions of the amygdala, orbital frontal cortex, temporal pole produce alteration of social behavior caused, in large part, by an incapacity to produce correct response to social stimuli [50]. In contrast to the 'understanding' based on the affective valence of the stimuli, the 'understanding' mediated by mirror neurons appears to be disjoint from emotional and vegetative responses. The meaning of the observed action does not result from the emotions it evokes, but from a matching of the observed action with the motor activity which occurs when the individual performs the same action.

Biological movement implies, by definition, a change in the relations of the acting individual with the external world. These changes are signalled by proprioception, vision, and in the case of transitive actions, by touch. The consequences, positive or negative, of the movements are also monitored by senses and remembered. When an individual emits a movement, he, usually, predicts its consequences. The movement representation in the cortical areas and the movement consequences are associated. In other words the movement has a meaning (e.g. 'grasp') and this meaning is represented by a specific cortical activation pattern. Mirror neurons show that this movement knowledge can be attributed to actions made by others. When an external stimulus evokes a neural activity similar to that which, when internally generated, represents a certain action, the meaning of the observed action is recognized because of the similarity between the two representations, the one internally generated during action and that evoked by the stimulus. It will be too long to speculate here how the individual recognizes his own movements from those generated by others or how the pictorial aspect of the hand, which does not belong to the acting individual, becomes associated with his movement. It is enough here to say that both these problems are not impossible to solve, theoretically. What is important to stress here is that the proposed mechanism is based on a purely observation/execution matching system. The affective valence of the stimuli, even if possibly present, does not play a role in this 'understanding' system. We will see in the next sections the importance of this point for understanding the development of the observation/execution matching system in man.

4.3. Observation/execution matching system in man

The presence of an observation/execution mechanism in monkey's premotor cortex suggests that a similar mechanism may exist also in man. To test this prediction we studied the excitability of the motor cortex in a group of normal human subjects [13]. The assumption underlying the experiment was that, if the observation of a movement activates the premotor cortex also in man, this activation should induce an enhancement of motor evoked potentials elicited by the magnetic stimulation of the motor cortex. The subjects were stimulated in four conditions: while they observed an experimenter grasping 3D-objects, while they looked at the same 3D-objects, while they observed an experimenter tracing geometrical figures in the air with his arm, and during detection of the dimming of a light. Motor evoked potentials were recorded from arm muscles.

The results showed a significant increase of the motor evoked potentials in the two conditions in which subjects observed movements. Furthermore, the increase was found only in those muscles that were active when the subjects executed the previously observed actions. Although it is premature to draw any firm conclusion on this last point, because only two types of movements were tested, nevertheless the obtained data strongly suggest that in man there is an observation/execution matching system similar to that found in the monkey premotor cortex.

Admitted that an observation/execution matching system exists in man, the next problem is to assess where it is located. A way to discover it is to examine in which brain structures regional blood flow (rCBF) changes occur during hand movement observation.

We recently addressed this problem using positron emission tomography [53]. The experiment was carried out at the Milan PET center (ISHSR). We used three experimental conditions: Object observation, Grasping observation and Object prehension. Object observation was used as a control condition. Images were analyzed by using statistical parametric mapping (SPM).

The most striking result of the experiment was the presence, in Grasping observation condition, of a highly significant activation in the posterior part of the left inferior frontal gyrus. This region corresponds to the rostral part of Broca's area as defined by Penfield and Roberts [43]. Other active regions were present in the occipital lobe and in the middle temporal gyrus. Although not significant with the SPM procedure, a comparison between Grasping observation and Object prehension showed an activation also of the cortex in the precentral gyrus. This activation might explain the findings obtained with magnetic stimulation.

Results, at least at first glance, in contrast with ours were obtained by Decety et al. [7] in an experiment in which they studied the rCBF changes in three conditions: Object inspection, Movement observation and Motor imagery. In all three conditions the subjects were presented with 3D-objects generated by a virtual reality system. The same system generated also the image of the hand grasping the objects in Movement observation condition. The results showed an activation of the premotor areas during motor imagery, but neither premotor nor frontal activation during movement observation. In this condition the activation concerned mostly the extrastriate visual areas.

The negative results obtained by Decety et al. are not completely surprising. The virtual reality technology, as used in their experiment, is unable to create a hand identical to a human hand, but only a schematic 'hand'. Since non-biological stimuli are ineffective in exciting F5 mirror neurons (see Figure 2), it is likely that in their experiment the cortical matching system was not activated. The moving object activated essentially visual areas and especially those involved in movement detection.

4.4. F5 and Broca's area. What is in common?

Homologies between cortical areas of different species are always difficult. They are even more difficult when one deals with speech areas, which might be unique to humans. In man, the frontal region related to speech (Broca's area), as outlined by electrical stimulation studies [40,43], is formed by areas 44 and 45 of Brodmann. Area 44 corresponds to area FCBm of von Economo [12], while area 45 corresponds to area FD γ. The first has basically an agranular structure, while in the second a granular layer is present. Von Bonin compared the premotor cortex of human, chimpanzee and macaque monkey brains [2]. This author adopted the lettering of Von Economo and recognized an area similar in architecture to FCBm in both the chimpanzees and monkeys. In the macaque monkey the location of FCBm is basically co-extensive with the area named F5 by Matelli et al. [33]. A similarity between human and monkey's FCBm was found also by Galaburda and Pandya [15] and, more recently by Petrides and Pandya [48]. They restricted however the homology only to that part of F5 that is located in the posterior bank of the arcuate sulcus. Finally, on the basis of hodological considerations Mesulam suggested that the ventral parts of inferior area 6 (F5) and area 45 are the areas which might be the homologue of the human frontal speech areas [36].

Taken together, all these data point to F5 as the area which might be the anatomical homologue of human Broca's area. Two major differences, however, come immediately to mind. First, in F5 there is a large hand area representation, while Broca's area is classically thought of as an area related to the control of musculature responsible for spoken word production. Second, F5 is an area receiving visual and somatosensory inputs, while Broca's area is mostly related to auditory input.

Although differences in somatotopic organization between F5 and Broca's area certainly exist, these differences are probably more in terms of the extension of the somatotopic fields and detailed representation of some movements, than in terms of gross somatotopy. In F5, in addition to the hand field there is also a large mouth-face field located laterally to the former [52]. It is very likely that in man this field has grown in relations to speech development and the great motor difficulties that speech poses. The fact remains, however, that a mouth field pre-exists speech in F5. Conversely, a hand field appears to exist in the Broca's region. If clinical evidence in this sense may be questioned because of the proximity of Broca's area to motor centers controlling arm movements, some recent PET data by Petrides and collaborators suggest that this is the case [1]. These authors recently showed that during execution of a sequence of self-ordered hand movements there was a highly significant activation of Broca's area. These data fit well with the findings, reported above, that a sector of Broca's area becomes active during grasping observation.

At this point the fundamental question is the following. Is there something in common between the 'mirror' functions present in both F5 and Broca's area and Broca's speech functions? In order to answer this question, let us briefly examine what might be the possible precursors of language in monkeys.

Vocalization in response to particular stimuli is common in non-human primates. It is usually maintained, however, that speech of man and monkey vocal responses are different phenomena. First of all the structures responsible for vocal calls and speech are different. The first are mediated primarily by the cingulate cortex together with diencephalic and brain stem structure [23,29]. The second depends essentially upon the activity of a circuit, formed by the classical Wernicke and Broca's areas, which are located on the dorsolateral cortical convexity. Secondly, the monkey vocalization is intimately related to emotional and instinctive behavior, whereas speech is not. Thirdly, speech is basically a one-on-one social interaction, while vocal calls of monkeys are not aimed to one specific individual [30].

These facts led many authors to conclude that speech depends on a uniquely human neural mechanism which evolved 'de novo' [25,39,56]. This statement appears to be undeniable if vocal calls and the structures underlying them are considered the precursors of speech. There is, however, another fascinating possibility recently proposed by Mc Neilage [30]. The main tenet of McNeilage's theory is that speech evolved when a 'continual mouth open-close alternation, the two phases of which are subject to continual articulatory modulation, was superimposed on the basic mammalian mode of sound generation – larynx based phonation. The open–close alternation relates to the syllable and the open and closed phases correspond to consonants and vowel, respectively. According to the theory the vocal communication, based on open–close mandibular alternation, evolved from other mandibular cyclicities such as for example the 'lipsmacks'. This faciovisual communicative gesture occurs in a wide variety of social circumstances, it is produced by both males and females and, most importantly, is accompanied by eye contact. Thus, in contrast with vocal calls, it shows the one-on-one social interactions that characterize speech.

Summing up, according to Mc Neilage's theory, speech had its origin not in primate vocal calls, but in the primate use of communicative gestures. The communicative modality for these gestures was initially visual. Only later in evolution the communicative gestures became associated with sounds. This fundamental step led to an enormous enrichment of primate communicative possibilities which, ultimately, culminated in the appearance of speech.

The data discussed in the present article fit well with the theory of McNeilage. In addition, they offer a more general explanation of why the communication system in primates developed in the dorsolateral cortex. These data show that inferior premotor cortex is endowed with the capacity of matching an observed action with an executed action and that, very likely, this mechanism is at the basis of monkey understanding of actions made by other individuals. If this conclusion is correct, the functional specialization of human Broca's area derives from an ancient mechanism related to production and understanding of motor acts. From this mechanism evolved, possibly in relation with the development of a more complex social life, first the capacity to make and interpret facial communicative gestures and, then, the capacity to emit and understand 'verbal gestures'. It is likely that the sophisticated capacity of movement analysis shown by mirror cells is at the basis of the evolutionary prevalence of the lateral motor system on the medial one, related to emotion, in becoming the main communication channel in higher primates and man.

Acknowledgements

The work was supported by the Human Frontier Science Program and by grants from CNR and MURST to G.R.

References

[1]   Bonda, E., Petrides, M., Frey, S. and Evans, A.C. Frontal cortex involvement in organized sequences of hand movements: evidence from a positron emission tomography study, *Soc. Neurosci. Abstr.*, (1994) 152.6.

[2]   von Bonin, G. Architecture of the precentral motor cortex and some adjacent areas. In P. Bucy (Ed.), *The Precentral Motor Cortex*, University of Illinois Press, Urbana, 1944, pp. 7–82.

[3]   Brothers, L. The social brain: a project for integrating primate behavior and neurophysiology in a new domain, *Concepts Neurosci.*, 1 (1990) 27–51.

[4]   Brothers, L., Ring, B. and Kling, A. Response of neurons in the macaque amygdala to complex social stimuli, *Behav. Brain Res.*, 41 (1990) 199–213.

[5]   Bruce, C., Desimone, R. and Gross, C.G. Visual properties of neurons in a polysensory area in superior temporal sulcus of the macaque, *J. Neurophysiol.*, 46 (1981) 369–384.

[6]   Cavada, C. and Goldman-Rakic, P.S. Posterior parietal cortex in rhesus monkey. II. Evidence for segregated corticocortical networks linking sensory and limbic areas with the frontal lobe, *J. Comp. Neurol.*, 287 (1989) 422–445.

[7]   Decety, J., Perani, D., Jeannerod, M., Bettinardi, V., Tadary, B., Woods, R., Mazziotta, J.C. and Fazio, F. Mapping motor representations with positron emission tomography, *Nature*, 371 (1994) 600–602.

[8]   Desimone, R., Albright, T.D., Gross, C.G. and Bruce, C. Stimulus-selective properties of inferior temporal neurons in the macaque, *J. Neurosci.*, 8 (1984) 2051–2062.

[9] di Pellegrino, G., Fadiga, L., Fogassi, L., Gallese, V. and Rizzolatti, G. Understanding motor events: a neurophysiological study, *Exp. Brain Res.*, 91 (1992) 176–180.

[10] Dum, R.P. and Strick, P.L. The origin of corticospinal projections from the premotor areas in the frontal lobe, *J. Neurosci.*, 11 (1991) 667–689.

[11] Dum, R.P. and Strick, P.L. Premotor areas: nodal points for parallel efferent systems involved in the central control of movement. In D.R. Humphrey and H.-J. Freund (Eds.), *Motor Control: Concepts and Issues. Dahlem workshop reports*, Wiley, Chichester, 1991, pp. 383–397.

[12] von Economo, C. *The Cytoarchitectonics of the Human Cerebral Cortex*, Oxford University Press, London, 1929.

[13] Fadiga, L., Fogassi, L., Pavesi, G. and Rizzolatti, G. Motor facilitation during action observation: a magnetic stimulation study, *J. Neurophysiol.*, 73 (1995) 2608–2611.

[14] Ferrigno, G. and Pedotti, A. ELITE: a digital dedicated hardware system for movement analysis via real-time TV-signal processing, *IEEE Trans. Biomed. Eng.*, BME-32, 11 (1985) 943–950.

[15] Galaburda, A.M. and Pandya, D.N. Role of architectonics and connections in the study of primate brain evolution. In E. Armstrong and D. Falk (Eds.), *Primate Brain Evolution*, Plenum, New York, 1982, pp. 203–216.

[16] Gallese, V., Murata, A., Kaseda, M., Niki, N. and Sakata, H. Deficit of hand preshaping after muscimol injection in monkey parietal cortex, *NeuroReport*, 5 (1994) 1525–1529.

[17] Gentilucci, M., Fogassi, L., Luppino, G., Matelli, M., Camarda, R. and Rizzolatti, G. Functional organization of inferior area 6 in the macaque monkey. I. Somatotopy and the control of proximal movements, *Exp. Brain Res.*, 71 (1988) 475–490.

[18] Gross, C.G., Rocha-Miranda, C.E. and Bender, D.E. Visual properties of neurons in the inferotemporal cortex of the macaque, *J. Neurophysiol.*, 35 (1972) 96–111.

[19] He, S.Q., Dum, R.P. and Strick, P.L. Topographic organization of corticospinal projections from the frontal lobe – motor areas on the lateral surface of the hemisphere, *J. Neurosci.*, 13 (1993) 952–980.

[20] Hepp-Reymond, M.-C., Hüsler, E.J., Maier, M.A. and Qi, H.-X. Force-related activity in two regions of the primate ventral premotor cortex, *Can. J. Physiol. Pharmacol.*, 72 (1994) 571–579.

[21] Jeannerod, M. The representing brain: neural correlates of motor intention and imagery, *Behav. Brain Sci.*, 17 (1994) 187–245.

[22] Jeannerod, M., Arbib, M.A., Rizzolatti, G. and Sakata, H. Grasping objects: the cortical mechanisms of visuomotor transformation, *Trends Neurosci.*, 18 (1995) 314–320.

[23] Jurgens, U. Primate communication: signalling, vocalization. In G. Adelman (Ed.), *Encyclopedia of Neuroscience*, Birkhauser, Boston, 1987.

[24] Kurata, K. and Tanji, J. Premotor cortex neurons in macaques: activity before distal and proximal forelimb movements, *J. Neurosci.*, 6(1986) 403–411.

[25] Lancaster, J. *Primate behavior and the emergence of human culture*, Holt, Rinehart Winston, New York, 1973.

[26] Leonard, C.M., Rolls, E.T., Wilson, F.A.W. and Baylis, G.C. Neurons in the amygdala of the monkey with responses selective for faces, *Behav. Brain Res.*, 15 (1985) 159–176.

[27] Luppino, G., Matelli, M., Camarda, R., Gallese, V. and Rizzolatti, G. Multiple representations of body movements in mesial area 6 and the adjacent cingulate cortex: an intracortical microstimulation study, *J. Comp. Neurol.*, 311 (1991) 463–482.

[28] Luppino, G., Matelli, M. and Rizzolatti, G. Cortico-cortical connections of two electrophysiologically identified arm representations in the mesial agranular frontal cortex, *Exp. Brain Res.*, 82 (1990) 214–218.

[29] MacLean, P.D. Introduction: perspectives on cingulate cortex in the limbic system. In B.A. Vogt and M. Gabriel (Eds.), *Neurobiology of Cingulate Cortex and Limbic Thalamus: a Comprehensive Handbook*, Birkhauser, Boston, 1993.

[30] MacNeilage, P.F. The frame/content theory of evolution of speech production, *Behav. Brain Sci.*, in press.

[31] Matelli, M., Camarda, R., Glickstein, M. and Rizzolatti, G. Afferent and efferent projections of the inferior area 6 in the macaque monkey, *J. Comp. Neurol.*, 251 (1986) 281–298.

[32] Matelli, M., Luppino, G., Murata, M. and Sakata, H. Independent anatomical circuits for reaching and grasping linking the inferior parietal sulcus and inferior area 6 in macaque monkey, *Soc. Neurosci. Abstr.*, 20 (1994) 404.4.

[33] Matelli, M., Luppino, G. and Rizzolatti, G. Patterns of cytochrome oxidase activity in the frontal agranular cortex of macaque monkey, *Behav. Brain Res.*, 18 (1985) 125–137.

[34] Matelli, M., Luppino, G. and Rizzolatti, G. Architecture of superior and mesial area 6 and of the adjacent cingulate cortex, *J. Comp. Neurol.*, 311 (1991) 445–462.

[35] Matsumura, M. and Kubota, K. Cortical projection of hand–arm motor area from postarcuate area in macaque monkey: a histological study of retrograde transport of horseradish peroxidase, *Neurosci. Lett.*, 11 (1979) 241–246.

[36] Mesulam, M.M. Large-scale neurocognitive networks and distributed processing for attention, language, and memory, *Ann. Neurol.*, 28 (1990) 597–613.

[37] Muakkassa, K.F. and Strick, P.L. Frontal lobe inputs to primate motor cortex: evidence for four somatotopically organized 'premotor' areas, *Brain Res.*, 177 (1979) 176–182.

[38] Mushiake, H., Inase, M. and Tanji, J. Neuronal activity in the primate premotor, supplementary, and precentral motor cortex during visually guided and internally determined sequential movements, *J. Neurophysiol.*, 66 (1991) 705–718.

[39] Myers, R.E. Comparative neurology of vocalization and speech: proof of a dichotomy, *Ann. New York Acad. Sci.*, 280 (1976) 745–757.

[40] Ojemann, G.A. Brain organization for language from the perspective of electrical stimulation mapping, *Behav. Brain Sci.*, 2 (1983) 189–230.

[41] Oram, M.W. and Perrett, D.I. Responses of anterior superior temporal poly-sensory (STPa) neurons to 'biological motion' stimuli, *J. Cogn. Neurosci.*, 6 (1994) 99–116.

[42] Passingham, R. *The Frontal Lobes and Voluntary Action*, Oxford, Oxford University Press, 1993, p. 299.

[43] Penfield, W. and Roberts, L. *Speech and Brain Mechanisms*, Princeton University Press, Princeton, 1959.

[44] Perrett, D.I., Harries, M.H., Bevan, R., Thomas, S., Benson, P.J., Mistlin, A.J., Chitty, A.K., Hietanen, J.K. and Ortega, J.E. Frameworks of analysis for the neural representation of animate objects and actions, *J. Exp. Biol.*, 146 (1989) 87–113.

[45] Perrett, D.I., Rolls, E.T. and Caan, W. Visual neurones responsive to faces in the monkey temporal cortex, *Exp. Brain Res.*, 47 (1982) 329–342.

[46] Perrett, D.I., Mistlin, A.J., Harries, M.H. and Chitty, A.J. Understanding the visual appearance and consequence of hand actions. In M.A. Goodale (Ed.), *Vision and Action: the Control of Grasping*, Ablex, Norwood, NJ, 1990, pp. 163–180.

[47] Petrides, M. and Pandya, D.N. Projections to the frontal cortex from the posterior parietal region in the rhesus monkey, *J. Comp. Neurol.*, 228 (1984) 105–116.

[48] Petrides, M. and Pandya, D.N. Comparative architectonic analysis of the human and the macaque frontal cortex. In F. Boiler and J. Grafman (Eds.), *Handbook of Neuropsychology*, Vol. IX, Elsevier, New York, 1994, pp. 17–58.

[49] Pigarev, I.N., Rizzolatti, G. and Scandolara, C. Neurons responding to visual stimuli in the frontal lobe of macaque monkeys, *Neurosci. Lett.*, 12 (1979) 207–212.

[50] Price, J.L., Russchen, F.T. and Amaral, D.G. The amygdaloid complex. In L.W. Swanson, A. Björklund and T. Hökfelt (Eds.), *Handbook of Chemical Neuroanatomy*, Elsevier, New York, 1987, pp. 279–388.

[51] Rizzolatti, G. Nonconscious motor images, *Behav. Brain Sci.*, 17 (1994) 220.

[52] Rizzolatti, G., Camarda, R., Fogassi, L., Gentilucci, M., Luppino, G. and Matelli, M. Functional organization of inferior area 6 in the macaque monkey. II. Area F5 and the control of distal movements, *Exp. Brain Res.*, 71 (1988) 491–507.

[53] Rizzolatti, G., Fadiga, L., Matelli, M., Bettinardi, V., Perani, D. and Fazio, F. Localization of cortical areas responsive to the observation of hand grasping movements in humans: a PET study, submitted.

[54] Rizzolatti, G., Gentilucci, M., Camarda, R., Gallese, V., Luppino, L., Matelli, M. and Fogassi, L. Neurons related to reaching-grasping arm movements in the rostral part of area 6 (area 6a β), *Exp. Brain Res.*, 82 (1990) 337–350.

[55] Rizzolatti, G., Scandolara, C., Gentilucci, M. and Camarda, R. Response properties and behavioural modulation of 'mouth' neurons of the postarcuate cortex (area 6) in macaque monkey, *Brain Res.*, 255 (1981) 421–424.

[56] Robinson, B.W. Limbic influences on human speech, *Ann. New York Acad. Sci.*, 280 (1976) 761–771.

[57] Sakata, H., Taira, M., Mine, S. and Murata, A. Hand-movement related neurons of the posterior parietal cortex of the monkey: their role in visual guidance of hand movements. In R. Caminiti, P.B. Johnson and Y. Burnod (Eds.), *Control of Arm Movement in Space, Exp. Brain Res., Suppl. 22*, Springer-Verlag, Berlin, 1992, pp. 185–198.

[58] Taira, M., Mine, S., Georgopulos, A.P., Murata, A. and Sakata, H. Parietal cortex neurons of the monkey related to the visual guidance of hand movement, *Exp. Brain Res.*, 83 (1990) 29–36.

[59] Weinrich, M., Wise, S.P. and Mauritz, K.M. A neurophysiological study of the premotor cortex in the rhesus monkey, *Brain*, 107 (1984) 385–414.

[60] Wise, S.P. The primate premotor cortex: past, present and preparatory, *Annu. Rev. Neurosci.*, 8 (1985) 1–19.

Appendix 3 – Chapter 4

Processing of illusion of length in spatial hemineglect: a study of line bisection

Vallar, G., Daini, R. and Antonucci, G. (2000)
Neuropsychologia, 38(7): 1087–97.

Abstract

Bisection of horizontal lines and of the Brentano form of the Müller-Lyer illusion was investigated in six right brain-damaged patients with left spatial hemineglect, and in six control subjects. Patients bisected the lines to the right of the objective mid-point. Comparable illusory effects on line bisection were however found in both patients and control subjects. Relative to the baseline condition, in both groups the subjective mid-point was displaced towards the side expanded by the illusion, both leftwards and rightwards. By contrast, line length and spatial position of the stimulus had differential effects. In neglect patients, the rightward bisection error increased disproportionately with line length, and when the stimulus was located in the left, neglected, side of egocentric space. Control subjects showed no such effects. The suggestion is made that the visual, non-egocentric, processes underlying these illusory effects of length may be spared in patients with left spatial neglect. The possible neural basis of this dissociation is discussed.

1. Introduction

A main and widely investigated manifestation of neglect for the contralesional side of space is the ipsilesional displacement of the subjective mid-point of a horizontal line in the bisection task. Right brain-damaged patients with left neglect set the perceived mid-point to the right of the objective centre of the segment [4,5,20,46,49].

A number of interpretations have been put forward to account for this rightward directional error. According to some early views, patients with unilateral neglect, due to a higher-order non-sensory disorder, fail to take into consideration the left side of the horizontal segment, or part of it, at least for the purpose of computing the subjective mid-point. Suggestions have been made that the left-to-right distribution of spatial attention may be defective, with the left side of the stimulus being comparatively less attended than the right [46]. The disorder may affect the internal representation of the stimulus, with a *representational scotoma* concerning the left side [4].

More recently, attempts have been made to elucidate in more detail the pathological mechanisms underlying the rightward bisection error made by patients with left neglect. These patients may perceive objects in extra-personal space in a disordered fashion, which primarily concerns their horizontal, left-to-right, extent. The left side, or part of it, might not be unattended, or its internal representation lost or cut, but *compressed* rightwards, with all spatially defined segments being available. Halligan and Marshall [19], who performed an experiment in which a right brain-damaged patient with left neglect was required to estimate visually the spatial position pointed to by an arrow, suggested that points in space may be pathologically compressed rightwards, equivalently throughout the horizontal range of the target. A related view is that patients with left neglect may suffer from a *shrinkage* or *compression* in size perception, which, however, is confined to, or affects disproportionately, the left, contralesional, half of the perceived space. Patients with left neglect may judge the left half of a horizontal line shorter than the right [39], and underestimate the horizontal extent of stimuli presented in the left side of their egocentric space [38].

The hypotheses of a rightward compression of visual space and of underestimation of the size of contralesional stimuli predict that visual illusions, which modify the perceived length of a line, affect the subjective mid-point set by both normal subjects and patients with left neglect. The size of the effect of illusions such as the Müller-Lyer might however be substantially reduced in patients, given its relationship to the length of the shaft [45]. More specifically, the hypothesis of a rightward compression of the stimulus throughout the whole range of the target [19] predicts a global reduction of the illusory effects. By contrast, the underestimation of the size of the contralesional part of the stimulus [38,39] would produce a non-symmetrical reduction of the illusory effects, due to the comparatively minor perceptual salience of the left side of the configuration in patients with left neglect.

To illustrate how a normal system could make errors analogous to those of patients with neglect, Watt [61] makes use of the Oppel–Kundt illusion, in which a horizontal extent divided by vertical bars appears longer than the undivided extent. In this study, we made use of the Brentano or combined form of the Müller-Lyer illusion [8], which makes one half of the line longer than the other. This version includes both ingoing and outgoing fins together, embedding two opposite Müller-Lyer illusions in the same configuration (Figure 1). The ingoing fins bring about an underestimation of the horizontal extent between their vertices, the outgoing fins an overestimation. Accordingly, one half of the horizontal segment appears longer than the other [43,45].

To elucidate the relationships between the modulation of the perceived length of the line induced by the illusion and the pathological mechanisms of spatial neglect, we investigated also the role of two other factors, which may affect the patients' performance in line bisection:

Table 1 Demographical and neurological features of six right brain-damaged patients[a]

Patient	Age/sex	Duration	M	VFD
RD	78/F	4	+	+
GM	79/M	2	+	+
ZB	83/F	3	+	−
LC	68/M	3	+	+
AC	70/M	3	+	−
FC	71/F	2	+	−

[a] M = motor; VFD = left visual half-field deficit; duration: length of illness (months); +/−: presence/absence of deficit.

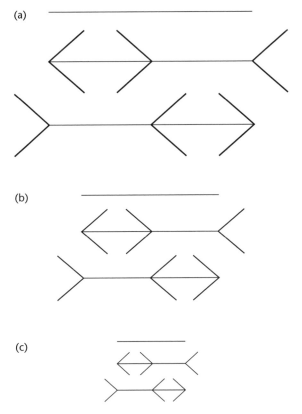

Figure 1 *Stimuli*. Simple line, and the Brentano form of the Müller-Lyer illusion with right-sided and left-sided outgoing fins for Experiments 1 and 2. (a), (b), and (c) show stimuli 24, 16, and 8 cm in length.

1. *line length*, with neglect patients making greater ipsilesional bisection errors with longer lines [4,17,34,42,46];
2. *spatial position of the stimulus* with reference to the egocentric frame of the mid-sagittal plane of the body, with patients making a minor error when the line is located in the right side of space, compared to centred or left-aligned conditions [7,20,27,35,49] (for a negative finding [46]).

2. Experiment 1

2.1. Materials and methods

2.1.1. Subjects

Six patients participated in the study. All patients were right-handed and showed no history or evidence of psychiatric disorders, or dementia. The patients' demographic

Table 2 Lesion localisation in five patients[a]

Patient	MFG	FO	FPR	preC	postC	SPL	IPL	TP	AC	supT	midT	postT	postGC	VAC	PVC
RD		x	x	x	x	x	x	x		x	x	x		x	
GM											x		x	x	x
ZB		x	x	x	x		x		x	x		x			
LC		x	x	x	x		x		x	x		x			
AC	x	x	x	x	x		x	x		x	x	x			(x)

[a] MFG (BA 46): middle frontal gyrus, dorsolateral prefrontal region; FO (BA 44, 45, 47): frontal operculum; FPR (BA 6): frontal premotor region; preC (BA 4): precentral gyrus; postC (BA 3, 1, 2): post-central gyrus; S/I PL (BA 7, 39 and 40): superior/inferior parietal lobule; TP (BA 38): temporal pole; AC (BA 41, 42): primary auditory cortex; supT (BA 22): superior temporal gyrus and auditory association cortex; midT (BA 21): middle temporal gyrus; postT (BA 37): posterior sector of middle, inferior and fourth temporal gyri; postGC (BA 23, 31): posterior half of cingulate gyrus; VAC (BA 18, 19): visual association cortex; PVC (BA 17): primary visual cortex; (x): minimal damage.

and neurological features are summarised in table 1. All patients showed evidence of left spatial neglect, as assessed by a standard diagnostic battery ([62] and below). Six right-handed subjects (mean age = 62.67 years, SD = 6.06, range = 54–68 years) with no history or evidence of neurological damage served as controls.

The side and the localisation of the cortico-subcortical lesions were assessed by CT or MRI, and analysed according to a standard method [10]. The lesion of patient FC was not mapped, due to the low quality of the MRI images, which prevented accurate analysis. Inspection of the images revealed an extensive cortico-subcortical ischaemic lesion in the vascular territory of the middle cerebral artery, involving the fronto-temporo-parietal cortex. Table 2 shows the localisation of the lesions in five patients. In four such patients the inferior parietal lobule, the superior temporal gyrus, the posterior sector of the middle and inferior temporal gyri, and the premotor and opercular frontal cortices were damaged. These findings are in line with previous anatomo-clinical correlation studies, suggesting that damage to the inferior parietal lobule [29,56], to the middle temporal gyrus and the temporo-parietal paraventricular white matter [48], and to the frontal opercular and premotor regions [23,56] brings about visuo–spatial neglect.

2.1.2.   *Baseline neuropsychological assessment*

A diagnostic battery, which included two visuo-motor exploratory tasks (line and letter cancellation), a reading task, and a task requiring a perceptual judgement assessed the presence of visuo–spatial neglect. In the cancellation tasks patients used the right hand. In all tasks the centre of the display was located on the mid-sagittal plane of the trunk of the patients, who were free to move their head and eyes [62]. All patients and control subjects had a normal or corrected-to-normal vision.

1. *Line cancellation* [1]. The scores were the numbers of omissions in the left- (range = 0–11) and right- (range = 0–10) hand sides of the sheet. Normal subjects perform this task without errors.
2. *Letter cancellation* [11]. The scores were the numbers of omissions on the left- (range = 0–53) and right- (range = 0–51) hand sides of the sheet. The maximum number of omission errors for normal subjects is four, and two is the maximum difference between errors on the two sides of the sheet [58].

Table 3 *Baseline assessment.* In the cancellation tasks (letter and line) the scores are the number of crossed targets, in the illusion test the number of unexpected responses, in the reading task the number of correctly read sentences

Test	Letter		Line		Illusion		Reading
Patient	Left	Right	Left	Right	Left	Right	
RD	0/53	29/51	7/11	10/10	19/20	0/20	0/6
GM	0/53	21/51	0/11	9/10	5/20	0/20	0/6
ZB	0/53	11/51	0/11	9/10	20/20	0/20	0/6
LC	19/53	43/51	0/11	8/10	19/20	0/20	0/6
AC	0/53	9/51	3/11	9/10	13/20	0/20	0/6
FC	5/53	26/51	3/11	10/10	4/20	0/20	2/6

3. *Sentence Reading.* The score was the number of incorrectly read sentences (range = 0–6). Normal subjects and patients with right brain damage without neglect make no errors on this test. Patients with left neglect make omission errors, substitution errors, or both, in the left half of the sentence.
4. *Wundt–Jastrow Area Illusion Test* [36]. The score was the number of responses not showing the illusory effect ('unexpected'), arising from the left (range = 0–20), and right (range = 0–20) sides of the stimulus. Patients with right brain damage and left neglect make errors only on stimuli with a left-sided illusory effect.

The results of the baseline neuropsychological assessment are summarised in Table 3. All patients showed evidence of left neglect in the four tasks.

2.1.3.   Stimuli and procedure

A Brentano version of the Müller-Lyer illusion was used [8]. The stimuli were printed on A4 sheets using two different colours for the fins (black) and the line (red). The stimuli included two experimental illusory conditions (*left-sided outgoing fin/right-sided ingoing fin*, and *left-sided ingoing fin/right-sided outgoing fin*), and a *baseline control condition* (*a red line*). Throughout the paper, the two types of illusory stimuli shall be distinguished with reference to the endpoint of the line (left or right) with the outgoing fin. Examples are shown in Figure 1. Three different line lengths were used for each condition (8, 16, and 24 cm). The fins were 2 cm long for 8 cm lines, 4 cm long for 16 cm lines, and 6 cm long for 24 cm lines. Lines and fins were 1 mm in width for 8 cm lines, 2 mm for 16 cm lines, and 3 for 24 cm lines. The fins formed with the line a 45° (ingoing) or 135° (outgoing) angle. Two blocks were generated. Block-A included the illusory stimulus with right-sided outgoing fin and the baseline stimuli (red line), block-B the left-sided outgoing fin and the baseline stimuli. Each block comprised 18 stimuli, with three trials for each of two conditions (illusory and baseline stimuli), for each of the three line lengths. Within each block the stimuli were presented in a random fixed order. Each block was presented twice according to an ABBA sequence. In each trial the centre of the stimulus was aligned with the mid-sagittal plane of the trunk of the subject. The subjects' task was to mark the mid-point of the red horizontal line, using a softpen, with no instructions about the fins being provided. All subjects used their right hand. Deviations from the objective midpoint of the red line were measured to the nearest millimetre. A positive score denoted a rightward transaction displacement, a negative score a leftward displacement.

These measures were submitted to a repeated measures analysis of variance with a between-subjects factor (*group*: patients and controls), and two within-subjects factors (*condition*: right-sided outgoing fin, left-sided outgoing fin, and simple line; *length*: 8, 16, 24 cm).

2.2. Results

Figure 2 shows the mean transaction errors (mm) of control subjects and patients with left neglect. The analysis of variance showed a main effect of the *group* factor $(F(1,10) = 6.3, P = 0.031)$, with neglect patients making a greater rightward transaction displacement. The main effect of *condition* was significant $(F(2,20) = 38.52, P < 0.0001)$. In both patients with neglect and control subjects the subjective mid-point was affected by the direction of the illusion: compared to the baseline control condition, right-sided outgoing fin stimuli brought about a rightward deviation, left-sided outgoing fin stimuli a leftward deviation. The main effect of *length* $(F(2,20) = 17.12, P < 0.0001)$, the *length* by *group* $(F(2,20) = 15.68, P < 0.0001)$ and the *condition* by *length* $(F(4,40) = 36.55, P < 0.0001)$ interactions were significant. Neither the *condition* by *group* $(F(2,20) = 1.97,$ n.s.$)$ nor the *condition* by *length* by *group* $(F(4,40) = 2.57,$ n.s.$)$ interactions attained a significant level. The effect of line length, as assessed by 8 vs 24 cm lines planned comparisons was significant in patients with neglect $(F(1,10) = 33.49, P = 0.00017)$, but not in control subjects $(F < 1,$ n.s.$)$.

The effects of *length* and *condition* and their interaction were further explored by two repeated measures analyses of variance, one in control subjects and one in patients with neglect, with two within-subjects factors.

In control subjects, the main effect of *condition* $(F(2, 10) = 158.51, P < 0.0001)$ and the *condition* by *length* interaction $(F(4,20) = 65.74, P < 0.0001)$ were significant, while the main effect of *length* was not $(F < 1,$ n.s.$)$. In the simple line condition minimal effects of line length were found. A Duncan's post-hoc test showed no significant differences between the mean bisection errors for 8 cm and 24 cm, and for 16 cm and 24 cm, with only the difference between errors for 8 and 16 cm being marginally significant $(P = 0.048)$. By contrast, in the two illusory conditions, the longer was the line, the greater the mean bisection error: for right-sided outgoing fin stimuli all differences between the mean errors for 8, 16 and 24 cm stimuli were significant $(P < 0.001)$; for left-sided outgoing fin stimuli the difference between the mean errors for 8 and 16 cm stimuli approached significance $(P = 0.061)$, with all other differences being significant $(P < 0.001)$. In all three line lengths both the left-sided and the right-sided outgoing fin conditions increased the magnitude of the bisection error relative to the simple line condition: all differences between mean errors were significant $(P < 0.001)$.

In patients with neglect, the main effects of *condition* $(F(2,10) = 15.51, P < 0.001)$, *length* $(F(2,10) = 16.52, P = 0.0007)$, and the *condition* by *length* interaction $(F(4,20) = 15.78, P < 0.0001)$ were significant. A Duncan's post-hoc test showed that in all three line

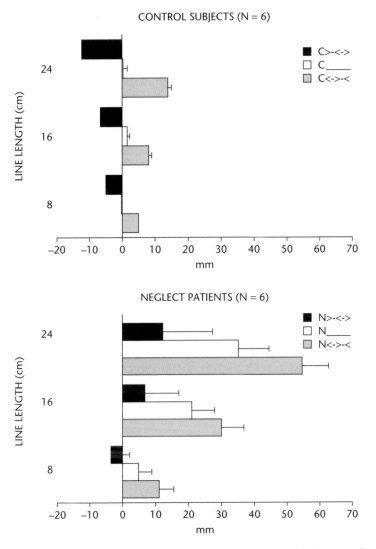

Figure 2 *Experiment 1.* Mean transaction displacements and standard errors of control subjects and patients with left hemineglect, by line length (8, 16, and 24 cm) and stimulus type (simple line, right-sided outgoing fin, left-sided outgoing fin).

lengths both the left-sided and the right-sided outgoing fin conditions increased the magnitude of the bisection error relative to the simple line condition: for 8 cm left- and right-sided outgoing fin stimuli the differences from the simple line were significant at $P < 0.05$; all other differences between mean errors were significant at $P < 0.01$. In both the simple line and the right-sided outgoing fin conditions all differences between 8, 16 and 24 cm stimuli were significant ($P < 0.0001$); in the left-sided outgoing fin condition the differences between the 8 and 16 cm, and the 8 and 24 cm stimuli were significant at $P < 0.0001$, the difference between 16 and 24 cm stimuli at

$P = 0.041$. As shown in Figure 2, the absolute increases of the rightward bisection errors were 16.14 mm (8 vs 16 cm lines) and 14.20 mm (16 vs 24 cm lines) for simple lines, 18.89 mm and 24.56 mm for right-sided outgoing fins, but comparatively minor (10.28 mm and 5.72 mm) for left-sided outgoing fins.

A perusal of the performance of the individual patients showed displacements of the subjective mid-point in the directions predicted by the illusory effects in five cases. Patient GM did not show the illusory effects with left-sided outgoing fins for 24 cm stimuli, with an increase of the rightward displacement error (+3.62 mm) relative to the simple line, and for 16 cm stimuli (−0.12 mm). A minor leftward effect was present for 8 cm stimuli (−1.67 mm, controls' mean = −4.96 mm, range = −7.79 to −2.54).

2.3. Discussion

The main result of this experiment is a dissociation between the average effects of the illusion, which were similar in the two groups, and those of line length, which were not. Both control subjects and patients with neglect showed average comparable effects of the two illusory conditions. In addition, in both groups the magnitude of the illusory effects increased with shaft length. This result is in line with previous observations in normal subjects, showing that in the Müller-Lyer figure the illusory effects are approximately proportional to shaft length [45].

In the simple line condition, by contrast, different effects of length were found in the two groups. In patients with neglect, the longer the line, the greater was the rightward transaction error, as found in many earlier studies (see Introduction). In control subjects the effects of line length were marginal, with the mean bisection errors being less than 1 per cent of total line length. A minor significant increase of the bisection error between 8 and 16 cm stimuli was found. Also the variability (standard error, mm) increased with line length (8 cm: 0.36; 16 cm: 0.98; 24 cm: 1.32). This pattern of performance of normal subjects replicates many previous observations [5,9,18,32,35,42].

Finally, in patients with neglect the quantitatively minor, albeit significant, effect of shaft length in the left-sided outgoing fin condition may reflect a performance compromise between the opposite effects of line length *per se*, on the one hand, which dramatically increases the rightward directional bias, and of the dimensions of the left-sided outgoing fin stimulus, on the other, which bring about a proportionally greater leftward shift. This would result in a comparatively minor length effect for left-sided outgoing fin stimuli.

3. Experiment 2

3.1. Materials and methods

3.1.1. Subjects

Patients were the same as in Experiment 1. Six new normal subjects (mean age = 68.33 years, SD = 7.2, range = 54–73 years) served as controls.

3.1.2. Stimuli and procedure

The stimuli and the bisection task were the same as in Experiment 1. This experiment differed from the previous one in that the effect of the position of the stimulus with respect to the mid-sagittal plane of the subject's body was investigated. Three positions of the line were assessed: (A: *centre*) the objective mid-point of the line was centred with respect to the mid-sagittal plane of the subject's trunk; (B: *left*) the right end-point of the line was aligned with the mid-sagittal plane of the trunk; (C: *right*) the left endpoint of the line was aligned with the mid-sagittal plane. Each block comprised 27 stimuli: three trials for each of the three conditions (line with right-sided outgoing fin, line with left-sided outgoing fin, simple line), for each of three line lengths (8, 16, and 24 cm). Within each block the stimuli were presented in a random fixed order. Each block was presented twice, in each of the three positions, according to an ABCCBA sequence. These measures were submitted to two repeated measures analysis of variance, one in control subjects and one in patients with neglect, with three within-subjects factors (*condition*: right-sided outgoing fin stimuli, left-sided outgoing fin stimuli, simple line; *length*: 8, 16, 24 cm; *position*: centre, left, right).

3.2. Results

The bisection performance of control subjects was affected by the illusory condition, confirming the results of the previous experiment, with no general effects of the spatial position of the stimuli (Figure 3). The main effect of *condition* was significant ($F(2,10) = 101$, $P < 0.0001$), while those of *position* and *length* did not attain the significance level ($F < 1$, n.s.). The *condition* $\times$ *position* ($F(4,20) = 5.66$, $P < 0.005$), the *condition* $\times$ *length* ($F(4,20) = 43.46$, $P < 0.0001$), and the *condition* $\times$ *position* $\times$ *length* ($F(8,40) = 6.67$, $P < 0.0001$) interactions were significant. The *position* $\times$ *length* interaction was not significant ($F < 1$, n.s.). A Duncan's post-hoc test showed that in all three line lengths and spatial positions both the left-sided and the right-sided outgoing fin conditions increased the magnitude of the bisection error relative to the simple line condition, with the differences between the means being significant at $P < 0.001$. For 24 cm lines, the leftward displacement produced by left-sided outgoing fins was minor in the left position, compared with both the right and the centre positions ($P < 0.0001$).

The patients' performance was affected by the illusory condition and by stimulus length – confirming the results of the previous experiment – and by the spatial location of the stimulus (Figure 4). In the right position the patients' rightward transaction error was minor. The main effects of *condition* ($F(2,10) = 14.00$, $P = 0.0013$), *position* ($F(2,10) = 13.36$, $P = 0.0015$) and *length* ($F(2,10) = 9.41$, $P = 0.005$) were significant. The *position* $\times$ *length* ($F(4,20) = 3.31$, $P = 0.031$) and the *condition* $\times$ *length* ($F(4,20) = 25.39$, $P < 0.0001$) interactions were significant, while the *condition* $\times$ *position* and the *condition* $\times$ *position* $\times$ *length* interactions were not ($F < 1$, n.s.).

The *condition* $\times$ *length* interaction was explored by a Duncan's post-hoc test. In the simple line and in the right-sided outgoing fin conditions the differences between the means of the three lengths were significant ($P < 0.001$). In the left-sided outgoing fin condition the differences between the means of the 8 cm and 16 cm, and of the 8 cm and 24 cm stimuli were significant ($P < 0.01$), while the difference between the means

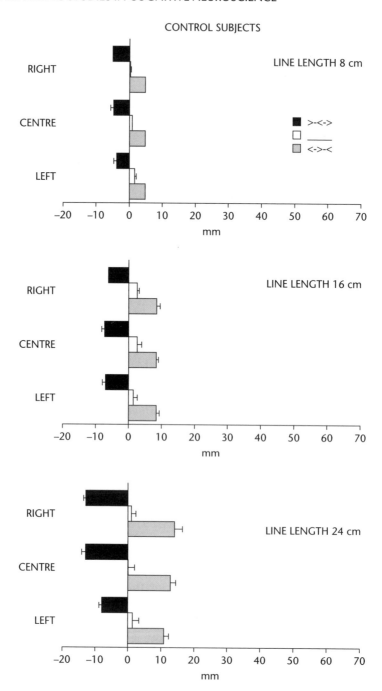

Figure 3 *Experiment 2. Control subjects.* Mean transaction errors and standard errors, by line length and stimulus type (see caption to Figure 2), and spatial position of the stimulus (right, centre, left).

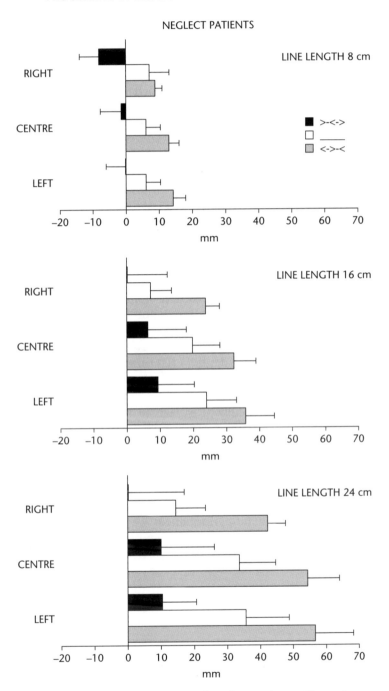

Figure 4 *Experiment 2 Patients with left hemineglect.* See caption to Figure 3.

of the 16 and 24 cm stimuli was not ($P=0.35$). Figure 4 shows in left-sided outgoing fin stimuli no increase of the rightward displacement from 16 to 24 cm; by contrast, in the other two conditions, the longer was the line, the greater the rightward directional error.

As for the *position* × *length* interaction, for each of the three stimulus lengths, significant differences ($P < 0.05$) between the means of the right and centre positions, and between the right and left positions were found. By contrast, the differences between the means of the centre and left positions were not significant. The differences between the three line lengths were significant in all three spatial positions ($P < 0.01$). Inspection of Figure 4 shows however that the effect of line length was minor in the right position, compared with both the centre and the left positions. Across conditions, the increases of the rightward displacement were 9.49 mm (8 vs 16 cm lines) and 9.08 mm (16 vs 24 cm lines) in the right position, 13.16 mm and 13.65 mm in the centre, 15.53 mm and 11.65 mm in the left position.

3.3. Discussion

The main result of this experiment is a dissociation in patients with neglect between the effects of the spatial position of the stimuli, and those of the illusory condition. Patients showed the illusory effects – confirming the results of the previous experiment – and their rightward transaction error was comparatively minor in the right position. These effects were however independent of each other. Again confirming the results of the previous study, the effect of shaft length for left-sided outgoing fin stimuli (16 vs 24 cm) was minor.

The performance of control subjects, as that of patients with left neglect, was affected by the illusory condition, but no general effects of stimulus length and spatial position were observed. The leftward displacement produced by the longest (24 cm) left-sided outgoing fin stimuli was however minor in the left position. With this type of stimulus the greatest leftward displacement of the subjective midpoint is the expected finding, and it is possible that the subjects' use of their right hand might have been a limiting factor. A complete assessment of this difference would require a study in which both left and right hand performances are assessed. This is an interesting issue in its own right, but in the present experiment the performance of normal subjects was meant to provide control data for the patients' scores, who used their right, non-paretic, hand.

4. General discussion

The rightward directional bias of the line bisection error of right brain-damaged patients with left spatial neglect is reduced, with a leftward displacement relative to the simple line condition, or increased, with a further rightward displacement, by a visual illusion which affects the perceived extent of a horizontal line. Similar illusory effects take place in normal subjects, whose bisection performance mimics left neglect, when the illusion brings about a reduction of the perceived horizontal extent of the left half of the line, compared with the right half. Conversely, a reduction of the perceived extent of the right half of the line produces a leftward displacement of the subjective mid-point, mimicking therefore neglect for the right side of the line. Fleming and Behrmann [13] have recently induced similar directional errors in normal subjects in a bisection task, using the Judd illusion, a variant of the Müller-Lyer illusion, that consists of an horizontal shaft with bilateral fins (see [31,44] for a discussion of the mechanisms underlying the illusory effects induced by the Judd and Müller-Lyer figures).

Two previous studies investigated the illusory effects of the Judd figure in patients with left spatial neglect. Ro and Rafal [47] found a dissociation between the defective perceptual awareness of the left-sided fins and the illusory effects of the stimulus (in both its left- and right-sided components) on the bisection performance of one right brain-damaged patient. Perceptual awareness was assessed by a discrimination task, in which the patient was required to decide whether or not two configurations producing the Judd illusion were identical or different (Patients with left neglect are typically unable to detect left-sided differences in a same-different judgement [6,33,57]). In a group of seven right brain-damaged patients with left neglect, Mattingley et al. [37] found consistent illusory effects with unilateral right and bilateral fin stimuli, with a leftward or rightward displacement of the perceived midline of the shaft. In the case of unilateral left fins, the illusory effects were less consistent across patients, but one case (No. 2) showed effects of both outward- and inward-projecting fins. In another patient (No. 1), however, both types of left-sided fins brought about a leftward displacement, reducing the bisection error. In cases of this sort the fins might have provided a summoning visual cue [16], without inducing any illusory effect. Both patients No. 1 and No. 2 were unable to report verbally the presence of left-sided fins, both in unilateral and bilateral fin configurations. Ro and Rafal [47], and Mattingley et al. [37] concluded that processes, perhaps preattentive, concerned with the appreciation of visual properties such as shape, could be undamaged in patients with left neglect, and underlie the displacements of the subjective mid-point induced by the illusion. Dissociations between inaccurate report and preserved effects of Gestalt grouping, producing Müller-Lyer illusory effects, have been found in normal subjects and interpreted with reference to differential contributions of attentional processes [40].

In the present study we attempted at dissociating the geometrical properties of the stimulus configuration, which underlie the illusory effects on length perception, from other characteristics of the stimulus, which, it has long been known, affect the bisection performance of patients with left spatial neglect. The disproportionate increase of the rightward bisection error with lines of increasing length found in patients with left neglect in Experiment 1, as well as in many previous studies, has been interpreted, in general terms, as resulting from a pathological orientation of spatial attention towards the rightmost extent of the stimulus line. According to one view [35], the bisection performance of normal subjects would reflect the ability to perform both left-to-right and right-to-left scantracks, from the leftmost and rightmost ends of the stimulus; patients with left neglect, by contrast, would confine their scans to a pathologically reduced right-to-left scan. In a computational model (MORSEL), which, after damage, simulates successfully the effects of line length on the bisection performance of patients with left neglect, the attentional mechanism component of the system is strongly biased towards the right portion of the line [42]. A mathematical model of line bisection in neglect also suggests a rightward bias of a salience-to-position curve [2]. Seen in this perspective, the dissociation found in patients with neglect between the pathological effects of line length, with a disproportionate increase of the bisection error, and the preserved effects of the illusion, suggests that these features of the stimulus probe the operation of independent systems. One view of accounting for the dissociation is in terms of a dysfunctional attentional system, pathologically biased towards the ipsilesional (right) endpoint of the stimulus, and non-attentional percep-tual processes, unaffected in patients with left neglect, which underlie the preserved illusory effects. In the present study, however, the dissociation did not contrast aspects of conscious perception, such as those assessed by same-different judgements [47] or verbal report [37], vs illusory effects, concerning instead the perceived horizontal extent of the stimulus. We therefore confine our conclusion to a dissociation between visual processes participating in the appreciation of the stimulus configuration, which underlie the illusory effects, and are preserved in the present series of patients with neglect, and a deranged system, pathologically sensitive to line length. This conclusion is corroborated by the recent report of a patient suffering from a selective dysmetrop-sia, yielding a disordered perception of size in the horizontal axis [14]. Patient P.S. showed a hemimicropsia, underestimating the size of objects presented in the left visual half-field, compared with objects presented in the right hemifield. P.S., however, showed no evidence of spatial neglect in both cancellation and line bisection tasks. This pattern suggests the possibility of a dissociation opposite to the one found in the present study.

The results of the second experiment, in addition to confirming the presence of illusory effects in patients with left neglect, elucidate their nature, with reference to the coordinate systems or reference frames in which they take place. The extent of the rightward bisection error was reduced, even though the patients' performance remained defective, when the stimulus was located in the right side of space, with reference to the mid-sagittal plane of the subject's body. This finding, which replicates previous observations, suggests that a disorder concerning the egocentric (with reference to the mid-sagittal plane of the body) coordinate frame contributes, at least in part, to the rightward error committed by patients with neglect in the line bisection task. The illusory effects, by contrast, not only were preserved in patients with left neglect, but also unaffected by the spatial position of the stimulus. This dissociation suggests that they take place at a non-egocentric level of representation of the stimulus. This pre-served representation, where the illusory effect is generated, may constitute an input to higher-order spatial systems. At this level of representation, in patients with left neglect a rightward bias, additive to the effect of the illusion, would take place. A number of studies in the somatosensory [41,50] and visual [26] domains suggest that the neglect-related components of defective awareness of tactile and visual stimuli (*sensory hemi-inattention*, using Heilman, Watson, and Valenstein's terminology [21]) concern a spatial, egocentric, level of representation. The more peripheral (somato-topic and retinotopic) sensory levels are, by contrast, largely preserved [53,54]. Studies with event-related potentials which show preserved early sensory processing in patients with left neglect support this conclusion [3,59].

In patients with left neglect the illusory effects were unaffected by spatial position, even when the whole stimulus was located in the *left* side of space, *neglected* with reference to the mid-sagittal plane of the body. This finding makes unlikely the possibility that the preserved illusory effects reflect a relatively normal processing of either the *right* side (when the stimulus is centred on the mid-sagittal plane), or the whole Brentano–Müller-Lyer figure (when the stimulus is placed to the right of the mid-sagittal plane). This conclusion is further supported by the finding that the spatial position of the stimulus is an effective manipulation in other respects, reducing the bisection error of patients with left neglect, when the stimulus is located on the right side.

The rightward error committed by patients with left neglect in the bisection task may be explained in terms of left-to-right compression of visual space [19], underestimation of the size of contralesional stimuli [15,38,39], rightward distortion of egocentric spatial representations and reference frames (translation or clockwise rotation: [24,55]), pathological rightward deployment of spatial attention [25,28]. These putative dysfunctions however take place at a level of visual representation, different from the one concerned with the illusion itself. At this latter level, features such as the dimension of the stimulus are adequately represented. In addition, the finding that in normal subjects the Brentano version of the Müller-Lyer illusion induces a pattern of bisection performance similar to that of patients with contralesional neglect (see also [13] for an investigation of the effects of the Judd illusion, in line with the present results) argues for the plausibility of a general interpretation of the bisection performance of patients with left neglect in terms of a relative compression of the left side of the line, associated with a relative expansion of the right side. This putative pathological compression does not, however, occur at the level of representation where the illusory effects (relative expansion and compression, yielding a 'neglect-like' directional bias in line bisection) are generated: these, as the present study shows, are preserved in patients with left neglect.

The conclusion that the illusory effects of the Brentano–Müller-Lyer figure and the rightward directional error made by patients with left neglect reflect the operation, and the dysfunction, of discrete processing systems and coordinate frames is, by and large, in line with current neuroanatomical knowledge.

In patients with neglect the lesion frequently involves the posterior-inferior parietal region, sparing the occipital cortex [52,53,56]. The anatomical localisation of the right hemisphere damage in the present group of patients is in line with these previous observations. The anatomical basis of the Müller-Lyer illusory effects is not clearly defined, but recent functional imaging studies have provided evidence that the perception of illusions such as Kanizsa's triangle is associated with activation in the occipital extra-striate cortex (V2 and possibly V3) [12,22]. In the present study patient GM, who in experiment 1 showed minor illusory effects with left-sided outgoing fin stimuli, had a lesion involving the association and primary visual cortices (Table 2). In patient P.S. the underestimation of visual stimuli presented in the left visual half-field was associated with an occipital stroke involving the right prestriate areas [14]. More specifically, a study in normal subjects, using luminance and colour contrasts, has suggested that geometric optical illusions of parallelness, length and size (Zollner, Müller-Lyer, Ponzo and Delboeuf) are mediated by the parvocellular system [30]. By contrast, a visual evoked potential study in right brain-damaged patients using visual stimuli modulated either in luminance or in chromaticity indicates that left neglect may be associated with a selective deficit to the magnocellular pathway [51]. This magno-dominated stream leads primarily to the posterior parietal cortex [60], which, as noted earlier, is a main anatomical correlate of unilateral neglect [52,53,56]. This evidence from neuroimaging, psychophysical, and neurophysiological studies in normal subjects and brain-damaged patients concurs therefore with the present results to suggest that discrete brain regions contribute to the representation of space, disrupted in patients with unilateral neglect, and to visual processes, such as the illusory perception of length.

Acknowledgements

This work was supported in part by grants from Ministero della Sanità, MURST and CNR.

References

[1]   Albert, M.L. A simple test of visual neglect. Neurology 1973;23:658–64.
[2]   Anderson, B. A mathematical model of line bisection behaviour in neglect. Brain 1996;119:841–50.
[3]   Angelelli, P., De Luca, M., Spinelli, D. Early visual processing in neglect patients: A study with steady-state VEPs. Neuropsychologia 1996;34:1151–7.
[4]   Bisiach, E., Bulgarelli, C., Sterzi, R., Vallar, G. Line bisection and cognitive plasticity of unilateral neglect of space. Brain and Cognition 1983;2:32–8.
[5]   Bisiach, E., Capitani, E., Colombo, A., Spinnler, H. Halving a horizontal segment: a study on hemisphere-damaged patients with cerebral focal lesions. Archives Suisses de Neurologie, Neurochirurgie et de Psychiatrie 1976;118:199–206.
[6]   Bisiach, E., Rusconi, M.L. Break-down of perceptual awareness in unilateral neglect. Cortex 1990;26:643–9.
[7]   Butter, C.M., Mark, V.W., Heilman, K.M. An experimental analysis of factors underlying neglect in line bisection. Journal of Neurology, Neurosurgery, and Psychiatry 1988;51:1581–3.
[8]   Coren, S., Girgus, J.S. Visual illusions. In: Held, R., Leibowitz, H.W., Teuber, H.-L. editors. Handbook of sensory physiology perception, Vol. 8. Heidelberg: Springer-Verlag, 1978. pp. 548–68.
[9]   D'Erme, P., De Bonis, C., Gainotti, G. Influenza dell'emi-inattenzione e dell'emianopsia sui compiti di bisezione di linee nei pazienti cerebrolesi. Archivio di Psicologia, Neurologia e Psichiatria 1987;48:193–207.
[10] Damasio, H., Damasio, A.R. Lesion analysis in neuropsychology. New York: Oxford University Press, 1989.
[11] Diller, L., Weinberg, J. Hemi-Inattention in rehabilitation. The evolution of a ra-tional remediation program. In: Weinstein, E.A., Friedland, R.P., editors. Hemiinattention and hemisphere specialization. New York: Raven Press, 1977. pp. 62–82.
[12] Ffytche, D.H., Zeki, S. Brain activity related to the perception of illusory contours. Neuroimage 1996;3:104–8.

[13] Fleming, J., Behrmann, M. Visuospatial neglect in normal subjects: altered spatial representations induced by a perceptual illusion. Neuropsychologia 1998;36:469–75.

[14] Frassinetti, F., Nichelli, P., di Pellegrino, G. Selective horizontal dysmetropsia following prestriate lesion. Brain 1999;122:339–50.

[15] Gainotti, G., Tiacci, C. The relationships between disorders of visual perception and unilateral spatial neglect. Neuropsychologia 1971;9:451–8.

[16] Halligan, P., Marshall, J.C. Right-sided cueing can ameliorate left neglect. Neuropsychological Rehabilitation 1994;4:63–73.

[17] Halligan, P.W., Marshall, J.C. How long is a piece of string? A study of line bisection in a case of visual neglect. Cortex 1988;24:321–8.

[18] Halligan, P.W., Marshall, J.C. Line bisection in visuo–spatial neglect: disproof of a conjecture. Cortex 1989;25:517–21.

[19] Halligan, P.W., Marshall, J.C. Spatial compression in visual neglect: a case study. Cortex 1991;27:623–9.

[20] Heilman, K.M., Valenstein, E. Mechanisms underlying hemispatial neglect. Annals of Neurology 1979;5:166–70.

[21] Heilman, K.M., Watson, R.T., Valenstein, E. Neglect and related disorders. In: Heilman, K.M., Valenstein, E., editors. Clinical neuropsychology. New York: Oxford University Press, 1993. p. 279–336.

[22] Hirsch, J., Delapaz, R.L., Relkin, N.R., Victor, J., Kim, K., Li, T., Borden, P., Rubin, N., Shapley, R. Illusory contours activate specific regions in human visual cortex. Evidence from functional magnetic-resonance-imaging. Proceedings of the National Academy of Sciences, USA 1995;92:6469–73.

[23] Husain, M., Kennard, C. Visual neglect associated with frontal lobe infarction. Journal of Neurology 1996;243:652–7.

[24] Karnath, H.-O. Spatial orientation and the representation of space with parietal lobe lesions. Philosophical Transactions of the Royal Society of London 1997;B352:1411–9.

[25] Kinsbourne, M. Orientational bias model of unilateral neglect: evidence from attentional gradients within hemispace. In: Robertson, I.H., Marshall, J.C., editors. Unilateral neglect: clinical and experimental studies. Hove: Erlbaum, 1993. pp. 63–86.

[26] Kooistra, C.A., Heilman, K.M. Hemispatial visual inattention masquerading as hemianopia. Neurology 1989;39:1125–7.

[27] Koyama, Y., Ishiai, S., Seki, K., Nakayama, T. Distinct processes in line bisection according to severity of left unilateral spatial neglect. Brain and Cognition 1997;35:271–81.

[28] Làdavas, E. Spatial dimensions of automatic and voluntary orienting components of attention. In: Robertson, I.H., Marshall, J.C., editors. Unilateral neglect: clinical and experimental studies. Hove: Erlbaum, 1993. pp. 193–209.

[29] Leibovitch, F.S., Black, S.E., Caldwell, C.B., Ebert, P.L., Ehrlich, L.E., Szalai, J.P. Brain-behavior correlations in hemispatial neglect using CT and SPECT: The Sunnybrook Stroke Study. Neurology 1998;50:901–8.

[30] Li, C.Y., Guo, K. Measurements of geometric illusions, illusory contours and stereo-depth at luminance and color contrast. Vision Research 1995;35:1713–20.

[31] Mack, A., Heuer, F., Villardi, K., Chambers, D. The dissociation of position and extent in Müller-Lyer figures. Perception and Psychophysics 1985;37:335–44.

[32] Manning, L., Halligan, P.W., Marshall, J.C. Individual variation in line bisection: a study of normal subjects with application to the interpretation of visual neglect. Neuropsychologia 1990;28:647–55.

[33] Marshall, J.C., Halligan, P. Blindsight and insight in visuo–spatial neglect. Nature 1988;336:766–7.

[34] Marshall, J.C., Halligan, P.W. When right goes left: an investigation of line bisection in a case of visual neglect. Cortex 1989;25:503–15.

[35] Marshall, J.C., Halligan, P.W. Line bisection in a case of visual neglect: psychophysical studies with implications for theory. Cognitive Neuropsychology 1990;7:107–30.

[36] Massironi, M., Antonucci, G., Pizzamiglio, L., Vitale, M.V., Zoccolotti, P.L. The Wundt-Jastrow illusion in the study of spatial hemi-inattention. Neuropsychologia 1988;26:161–6.

[37] Mattingley, J.B., Bradshaw, J.L., Bradshaw, J.A. The effects of unilateral visuospatial neglect on perception of Müller-Lyer illusory figures. Perception 1995;24:415–33.

[38] Milner, A.D., Harvey, M. Distortion of size perception in visuospatial neglect. Current Biology 1995;5:85–9.

[39] Milner, A.D., Harvey, M., Roberts, R.C., Forster, S.V. Line bisection errors in visual neglect: misguided action or size distortion? Neuropsychologia 1993;31:39–49.

[40] Moore, C.M., Egeth, H. Perception without attention: evidence of grouping under conditions of inattention. Journal of Experimental Psychology: Human Perception and Performance 1997;23:339–52.

[41] Moscovitch, M., Behrmann, M. Coding of spatial information in the somatosensory system: evidence from patients with neglect following parietal lobe damage. Journal of Cognitive Neuroscience 1994;6:151–5.

[42] Mozer, M.C., Halligan, P.W., Marshall, J.C. The end of the line for a brain-damaged model of unilateral neglect. Journal of Cognitive Neuroscience 1997;9:171–90.

[43] Porac, C. Comparison of the wings-in, wings-out, and Brentano variants of the Müller-Lyer illusion. American Journal of Psychology 1994;107:69–83.

[44] Post, R.B., Welch, R.B., Caufield, K. Relative spatial expansion and contraction within the Müller-Lyer and Judd illusions. Perception 1998;27:827–38.

[45] Restle, F., Decker, J. Size of the Müller-Lyer illusion as a function of its dimensions: theory and data. Perception and Psychophysics 1977;21:489–503.

[46] Riddoch, M.J., Humphreys, G.W. The effect of cueing on unilateral neglect. Neuropsychologia 1983;21:589–99.

[47] Ro, T., Rafal, R.D. Perception of geometric illusions in hemispatial neglect. Neuropsychologia 1996;34:973–8.

[48] Samuelsson, H., Jensen, C., Ekholm, S., Naver, H., Blomstrand, C. Anatomical and neurological correlates of acute and chronic visuospatial neglect following right hemisphere stroke. Cortex 1997;33:271–85.

[49] Schenkenberg, T., Bradford, D.C., Ajax, E.T. Line bisection and unilateral visual neglect in patients with neurologic impairment. Neurology 1980;30:509–17.

[50] Smania, N., Aglioti, S. Sensory and spatial components of somaesthetic deficits following right brain damage. Neurology 1995;45:1725–30.

[51] Spinelli, D., Angelelli, P., De Luca, M., Burr, D.C. VEP in neglect patients have longer latencies for luminance but not for chromatic patterns. NeuroReport 1996;7:815–9.

[52] Vallar, G. The anatomical basis of spatial hemineglect in humans. In: Robertson, I.H., Marshall, J.C., editors. Unilateral neglect: clinical and experimental studies. Hove: Lawrence Erlbaum, 1993. pp. 27–59.

[53] Vallar, G. Spatial frames of reference and somatosensory processing: a neuro-psychological perspective. Philosophical Transactions of the Royal Society of London 1997;B352:1401–9.

[54] Vallar, G., Bottini, G., Rusconi, M.L., Sterzi, R. Exploring somatosensory hemi-neglect by vestibular stimulation. Brain 1993;116:71–86.

[55] Vallar, G., Guariglia, C., Nico, D., Bisiach, E. Spatial hemineglect in back space. Brain 1995;118:467–72.

[56] Vallar, G., Perani, D. The anatomy of unilateral neglect after right hemisphere stroke lesions. A clinical CT/Scan correlation study in man. Neuropsychologia 1986;24:609–22.

[57] Vallar, G., Rusconi, M.L., Bisiach, E. Awareness of contralesional information in unilateral neglect: effects of verbal cueing, tracing and vestibular stimulation. In: Umiltà, C., Moscovitch, M., editors. Attention and performance XV. Conscious and nonconscious information processing. Cambridge, Mass: MIT Press, 1994. pp. 377–91.

[58] Vallar, G., Rusconi, ML., Fontana, S., Musicco, M. Tre test di esplorazione visuo-spaziale: taratura su 212 soggetti normali. Archivio di Psicologia, Neurologia e Psichiatria 1994;55:827–41.

[59] Vallar, G., Sandroni, P., Rusconi, M.L., Barbieri, S. Hemianopia, hemianesthesia and spatial neglect. A study with evoked potentials. Neurology 1991;41:1918–22.

[60] Van Essen, D.C., Deyoe, E.A. Concurrent processing in the primate visual cortex. In: Gazzaniga, M.S., editor. The cognitive neurosciences. Cambridge, Mass: MIT Press, 1995. p. 383–100.

[61] Watt, R. Some points about human vision and visual neglect. Neuropsychological Rehabilitation 1994;4:213–9.

[62] Zoccolotti, P., Antonucci, G., Judica, A., Montenero, P., Pizzamiglio, L., Razzano, C. Incidence and evolution of the hemi-neglect disorder in chronic patients with unilateral right brain-damage. International Journal of Neuroscience 1989;47:209–16.

Appendix 4 – Chapter 5

A spelling device for the paralysed

Birbaumer, N., Ghanayim, N., Hinterberger, T., Iversen, I., Kotchoubey, B., Kübler, A., Perelmouter, J., Taub, E. and Flor, H. (1999)
Nature, 398: 297–8.

When Jean-Dominique Bauby suffered from a cortico-subcortical stroke that led to complete paralysis with totally intact sensory and cognitive functions, he described his experience in *The Diving-Bell and the Butterfly*[1] as 'something like a giant invisible diving-bell holds my whole body prisoner'. This horrifying condition also occurs as a consequence of a progressive neurological disease, amyotrophic lateral sclerosis, which involves progressive degeneration of all the motor neurons of the somatic motor system. These 'locked-in' patients ultimately become unable to express themselves and to communicate even their most basic wishes or desires, as they can no longer control their muscles to activate communication devices. We have developed a new means of communication for the completely paralysed that uses slow cortical potentials (SCPs) of the electroencephalogram to drive an electronic spelling device.

The neurophysiological basis and behavioural functions of SCPs have been described[2], and operant conditioning has been used to bring them under voluntary control. We have shaped the voluntary control of SCPs in two locked-in patients with amyotrophic lateral sclerosis who were able to learn to operate a spelling device by regulating their brain responses. The spelling device drives a cursor on a video screen, allowing the subjects to select letters of the alphabet. Previous interfaces between brains and computers have used different brain responses, such as certain frequency bins or event-related brain potentials[3,4], but these have not yet been tested with locked-in patients.

Both subjects suffer from advanced amyotrophic lateral sclerosis and have been artificially respirated and fed for four years. Sustained voluntary control of the musculature was not possible in either patient, so they were unable to use a muscle-driven communication device. They were trained to produce changes voluntarily in their SCPs lasting 2–4 seconds. Each trial consisted of a 2-second baseline and a response period lasting 2–4 seconds, the length of which was adapted to suit the patient. A training day consisted of 6–12 sessions (depending on the condition of the patient), each of which comprised about 70 to 100 trials and lasted about 5–10 minutes.

During the response period, the subjects were required to produce either negativity or positivity greater than a specific criterion amplitude in random order. The baseline and response periods were signalled by two clearly different tones, and whether positivity or negativity was required was indicated by a box being highlighted in either the upper (negativity) or the lower (positivity) half of the screen. Visual feedback of SCPs, which was updated every 64 ms, was provided by a ball that moved towards or away from the box, depending on the direction in which the SCP deviated from baseline. The response criterion was progressively increased from 5 to 8 μV.

SCPs were extracted from the regular electroencephalogram using a time constant of 8 s and a low-pass filter of 40 Hz. They were recorded from the vertex relative to linked mastoids at a sampling rate of 256 Hz. Vertical eye movements were simultaneously recorded with standard on-line removal of eye-movement artefacts[2]. Using an imagery strategy[5], both patients were better able to produce positivity than negativity, so training for negativity was soon discontinued. As soon as a stable performance of at least 75 per cent correct (hitting the goal for at least 500 ms) responses at the 8-μV level was achieved, the patients began to work with the spelling device. Subject A achieved this level after 327 sessions and subject B achieved it after 288 sessions (Figure 1).

For the spelling program at level 1, the alphabet was split into two halves (letter banks) which were presented successively at the bottom of the screen for 4.5 seconds (subject A) or 6 seconds (subject B). If the subject selected the letter bank being shown by generating a SCP, it was split into two new halves, and so on until each of the two letter banks had only one letter in it. When one of the two final letters was selected, it was displayed in the top text field of the screen and then the selection began again at level 1. A 'go back' function, which appeared as an option when two successive letter banks had not been selected, allowed the speller to go back one step to the previous set of letter banks. If the speller was at level 1, selecting this function erased the last symbol written in the text field, so mistakes could be corrected. This procedure was chosen after extensive pilot work[6] involving different types of speller.

The accuracy of responses during feedback training, copy spelling and free spelling is shown in Figure 1 for both patients over the course of 446 (subject A) and 308 sessions (subject B). Two types of error were possible: incorrect rejection was due to the SCP amplitude being too low, and incorrect selection occurred when a high SCP was made in the presence of a wrong letter or row of letters. Both subjects can now write messages. The first full message written entirely by the brain of subject A is shown in Figure 2.

Our data indicate that patients who lack muscular control can learn to control variations in their SCPs sufficiently accurately to operate an electronic spelling device. Although writing sentences is time consuming – subject A took 16 hours to write the message in Figure 2, a rate of about 2 characters per minute – it is reliable and precise enough to allow the patient to communicate with his or her environment. These completely paralysed individuals now have the ability to communicate, a possibility that has not previously existed for such severely affected patients.

Insect antenna as a smoke detector

The larvae of jewel beetles of the genus *Melanophila* (Buprestidae) can develop only in the wood of trees freshly killed by fire[1]. To arrange this, the beetles need to approach forest fires from as far as 50 kilometres away[1,2]. They are the only buprestid beetles known to have paired thoracic pit organs[3], which behavioural[2], ultrastructural[4] and physiological experiments[5] have shown to be highly sensitive infrared receptors, useful for detecting forest fires. It has been suggested that *Melanophila* can sense the smoke from fires[6], but behavioural experiments failed to show that crawling beetles approach

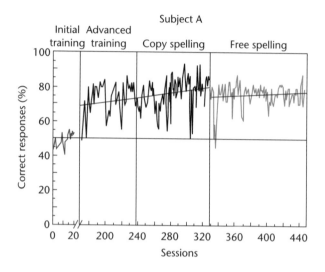

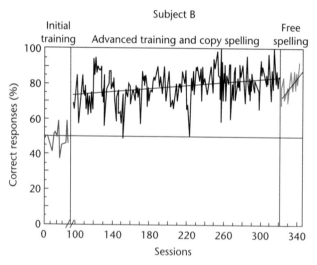

Figure 1 Response accuracy of subjects using the new spelling device. Subject A began with feedback training of SCP amplitude (initial and advanced training; 71.3% correct selections, 75.0% correct rejections, based on 'go-back' responses), proceeded to copy spelling (copying of letters and then words; 78.7%, 75.3%) and finally to free spelling (self-selected letters; 66.4%, 82.9%). Subject B began with initial training, then switched to a combination of advanced training (77.5%, 68.8%) and copy spelling (77.5%, 67.6%) and finally to free spelling (86.2%, 73.7%).

smoke sources[2]. We find that the antennae of jewel beetles can detect substances emitted in smoke from burning wood.

We connected freshly excised antennae from *M. acuminata* ($n = 5$) to a gas chromatograph equipped with parallel flame ionization and electroantennographic detectors[7]. Volatiles generated by smouldering splint wood from *Pinus sylvestris* were

LIEBER-HERR-BIRBAUMER-

HOFFENTLICH-KOMMEN-SIE-MICH-BESUCHEN,-WENN-DIESER-
BRIEF-SIE-ERREICHT-HAT-.ICH-DANKE-IHNEN-UND-IHREM-
TEAM-UND-BESONDERS-FRAU-KÜBLER-SEHR-HERZLICH,-DENN-
SIE-ALLE-HABEN-MICH-ZUM-ABC-SCHÜTZEN-GEMACHT,-DER-
OFT-DIE-RICHTIGEN-BUCHSTABEN-TRIFFT.FRAU-KÜBLER-IST-EINE-
MOTIVATIONSKÜNSTLERIN.OHNE-SIE-WÄRE-DIESER-BRIEF-NICHT-
ZUSTANDE-GEKOMMEN.-ER-MUSS-GEFEIERT-WERDEN.-DAZU-
MÖCHTE-ICH-SIE-UND-IHR-TEAM-HERZLICH-EINLADEN-.
EINE-GELEGENHEIT-FINDET-SICH-HOFFENTLICH-BALD.

MIT-BESTEN-GRÜSSEN-
IHR-HANS-PETER-SALZMANN

Figure 2 The first full message written by subject A.

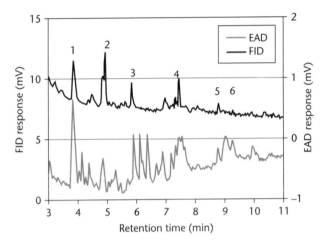

Figure 3 Typical gas chromatograms. Two detectors were used: a flame-ionization detector (FID), indicating any oxidizable compound; and an electroantennographic detector (EAD), using an isolated antenna of *Melanophila acuminata*. The sample contains volatiles released by 1 g of smouldering wood in 1 s, a quantity typically transported over long distances. The FID response indicates quantities of the mixture's components. The EAD response (amplified by a factor of 100) indicates the electrophysiological response of the antenna to: 1, α-pinene; 2, carene; 3, 2-methoxy-phenol (guaiacol); 4, 2-methoxy-4-methyl-phenol (4-methyl-guaiacol); 5, 4-acetyl-guaiacol; 6, 4-formyl-guaiacol. The two peaks only in the EAD trace (retention times of 6.0 to 6.5 min) indicate substances detected by antennae at concentrations below the detection limit of the FID: (10 ng per ml of carrier gas); presumably they are isomers of compound 3.

collected on a charcoal trap, chemodesorbed by an organic solvent, and injected into the apparatus. The resulting chromatograms indicated that several components of these volatiles were biologically active (Figure 3). Most of the volatiles perceived by the antennae are phenolic compounds, derivatives of 2-methoxyphenol (guaiacol) eliciting the greatest response.

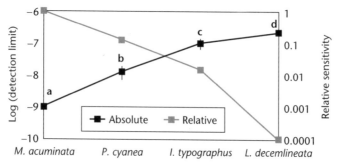

Figure 4 Absolute and relative sensitivities of pyrophilic and non-pyrophilic insects to guaiacol. Absolute detection limits were estimated by fitting logistic curves to dose-response data. The concentrations where confidence intervals (at 0.05) of average control responses did not overlap with confidence belts of fit functions were regarded as the limits of detection. Error bars show standard deviations. Letters indicate significantly differing responses (Mann-Whitney U test, $P < 0.05$) to concentrations at detection limits. For insects infesting pine trees, α-pinene was chosen as a reference substance for obtaining relative sensitivities, as it is a typical constituent of host plant odour with a low detection limit. (Z)-3-hexen-1-ol was chosen for the Colorado potato beetle (*L. decemlineata*) as a sensitively detected constituent of its host plant odour.

Methoxylated phenols are released by the incomplete combustion of lignin[8] and have been identified as atmospheric markers of wood smoke. The chemical structure of the phenolic compounds in smoke is dependent on the species of tree attacked by fire[9]. Because it is particularly sensitive to guaiacol derivatives, *Melanophila* can detect remote forest fires and might even be able to use the pattern of volatiles to identify the species of tree. Our results therefore indicate that the beetles can perceive a fire-damaged *P. sylvestris* tree by olfactory cues.

The beetles' antennae can detect these guaiacol derivatives at concentrations as low as a few parts per billion (p.p.b.) (Figure 4). We estimate[10] that this sensitivity is sufficient for the beetle to detect a single pine tree 30 cm in diameter that has smouldering bark to a height of 2 m and a bark depth of 1 cm, releasing about 7 g of guaiacol in an hour under light wind conditions (0.3 m s^{-1}), from a distance of more than 1 km.

M. acuminata shows a high absolute (1.1 ± 0.8 pg ml^{-1}, $n = 14$) and relative sensitivity to guaiacol. For comparison, we also studied the sensitivity to guaiacol of three other beetles. The pulp-feeding forest pest *Phaenops cyanea* attacks weakened trees and sometimes breeds in trees that have previously been damaged by fire. It is closely related to *M. acuminata*, but its attraction to fire-damaged trees is less pronounced. Its sensitivity to guaiacol is slightly lower at 15 ± 7 pg ml^{-1} ($n = 11$). The bark beetle *Ips typographus* is a pulp-feeding forest pest without detectable attraction to fire-damaged trees, but some sensitivity to guaiacols is expected because pulp also contains guaiacol. It shows only a moderate absolute (120 ± 65 pg ml^{-1}, $n = 9$) and relative sensitivity to this compound. The Colorado potato beetle, *Leptinotarsa decemlineata*, is a non-pyrophilic pest that is not attracted to fire-damaged trees, although it exhibits escape behaviour in response to high concentrations of fire-generated volatiles. It does not show such specialized sensitivity (450 ± 160 pg ml^{-1}, $n = 24$) to guaiacol derivatives. These values reflect the relative degree of specialization to fire detection.

In the same way that infrared-sensitive pit vipers and boid snakes use chemoreceptors on their tongue to detect volatiles released by their prey, *Melanophila* beetles use chemoreceptors sensitive to the specific volatiles of burning wood. It is unclear how the two sensory systems used by *Melanophila* to identify fire – the thoracic infrared receptors and the antennal olfactory receptors – act together to detect fire and orientate the beetle towards its source.

Understanding how the beetles detect fires could have applications in fire detection devices[11] in storehouses and public buildings, for example, as well as in early-warning detection systems for forest fires.

References

1. Bauby, J.-D. *The Diving-Bell and The Butterfly* (Fourth Estate, London, 1997).
2. Birbaumer, N., Elbert, T., Canavan, A.G.M. and Rockstroh, B. *Rhys. Rev.* **70**, 1–41 (1990).
3. Vaughan, T.M., Wolpaw, J.R. and Donchin, E. *IEEE Trans. Rehab. Eng.* **4**, 425–430 (1996).
4. Farwell, L.A. and Donchin, E. *Electroencephalogr. Clin. Neurophysiol.* **70**, 510–523 (1988).
5. Roberts, L.E., Birbaumer, N., Rockstroh, B., Lutzenberger, W. and Elbert, T. *Psychophysiology* **26**, 392–403 (1989).
6. Perelmouter, J., Kotchoubey, B., Kübler, A., Taub, E. and Birbaumer, N. *Automedica* (in the press).

Appendix 5 – Chapter 6

Non-conscious recognition of affect in the absence of striate cortex

de Gelder, B., Vroomen, J., Pourtois, G., and Weiskrantz, L. (1999) *Neuroreport*, 10(8): 3759–63.

Functional neuroimaging experiments have shown that recognition of emotional expressions does not depend on awareness of visual stimuli and that unseen fear stimuli can activate the amygdala via a colliculopulvinar pathway. Perception of emotional expressions in the absence of awareness in normal subjects has some similarities with the unconscious recognition of visual stimuli which is well documented in patients with striate cortex lesions (blindsight). Presumably in these patients residual vision engages alternative extra-striate routes such as the superior colliculus and pulvinar. Against this background, we conjectured that a blindsight subject (GY) might recognize facial expressions presented in his blind field. The present study now provides direct evidence for this claim. *NeuroReport* 10:3759–3763 © 1999 Lippincott Williams & Wilkins.

Key words: Awareness; Blindsight; ERPs; Facial expression; P1

Introduction

Evidence about the absence of conscious awareness in processing emotional information has emerged recently from a number of areas. Neuroimaging studies have shown amygdala activation to emotional stimuli, most notably to fearful faces [1,2]. Subcortical reactions to emotional stimuli have also been registered when stimulus awareness was prevented by backward visual masking of the emotional stimuli [3], including in a fear conditioning paradigm [4]. A prosopagnosic patient unable to recognize facial expressions as a consequence of focal brain damage in the occipito-temporal areas nevertheless showed a sizable impact of facial expressions on recognition of voice affect [5]. Such studies share a similarity with reports of processing of elementary visual stimuli in the absence of awareness in patients with striate cortex lesions (blindsight). These patients can make accurate guesses about the attributes of stimuli presented to their blind field of which they have no awareness.

The pathways of retinal origin that are most likely to be engaged by visual processing in the absence of striate cortex are the superior colliculus and the pulvinar. Neuroimaging studies [4] have provided evidence for selective involvement of these structures in conscious *vs* non-conscious recognition of facial expressions. Thus far, studies of residual visual abilities in patients with blindsight have mostly investigated covert perception of elementary visual information such as presence of a spatial frequency grating, discrimination of simple shape (such as O *vs* X) [6], detection of orientation or of direction of movement [7] or of colour [8–11]. Recently blindsight has been reported for some high level vision stimuli such as words [12]. Given the existence of alternative visual pathways that remain after loss of the pathway to striate cortex with data from studies showing non-conscious processing of emotional information, we conjectured that there might exist non-conscious recognition of facial expressions in such a case.

Here we report the first study of recognition of unseen emotional stimuli in a well-studied 43-year-old blindsight subject, GY (see [13] for a recent list of studies with GY and details about the lesion), who has a right half-field of blindness as a result of damage to his left occipital lobe at the age of 8. Behavioural methods were used to test whether he could discriminate different facial expressions and, if so, whether his good performance reflected covert recognition of the facial expressions rather than discrimination of two patterns of movement, and whether the actual conscious content of the alternative response labels he was given were important for his performance. As a follow-up we provide evidence for visual processing in the blind field obtained with event related potentials (ERPs).

Materials and Methods

Stimuli and tasks: Stimuli consisted of four video fragments showing a female face pronouncing the same sentence with four different facial expressions (happy, sad, angry, fearful). These materials were subsequently used in different presentation conditions. Presentation was either random between left/right visual fields or blocked, the image size could either be small ($10.2 \times 8.2°$) or large ($12.5 \times 10.7°$), and depending on the experiment the forced choice alternatives were either happy *vs* sad, or angry *vs* fearful. Mean luminance of the screen in between stimulus presentations was 1.5 cd/m^2. Mean luminance of the face was 20 cd/m^2 and for the grey frame around the image was 21 cd/m^2. Horizontal separation between the fixation point and the outer edge of the face was $3.6°$, for the eye it was $5.1°$, and for the center of the face it was $6.4°$. Stimulus duration was 1.63 s. All of the responses were made verbally.

In the first experiment a total of 8 blocks were run using different stimulus pairs (happy/sad, angry/sad, angry/fearful), different stimulus sizes (small or big), and different presentation conditions (randomized over left (LVF) or right (RVF) visual fields, or in blocks of trials to either field). In the second experiment, four different video fragments (happy/sad/angry/fearful) were presented in a four-alternative forced-choice design and shown in the RVF. They were presented randomly in two blocks of 72 trials each (18×4 categories). Instructions specified to label the videos as happy, sad, angry or fearful. The duration of each was 1.63 s. In the third experiment, all stimuli were the small size happy/fear faces, with presentation blocked or randomized. In the fourth experiment, The videos were of the same small-sized moving videos as described before with a $6.4°$ horizontal separation between the fixation point and the centre of the face. All videos were presented in the right visual field with the sound off, in blocks of 60 trials, 30 for each of the two categories being used (happy/sad or angry/fearful).

The categories were presented in random order. The two blocks with congruent labels were presented first (first happy/sad, then angry/fearful), and they were followed by the two blocks with non-congruent labels (first angry/fearful videos with happy/sad labels, then happy/sad videos with angry/fearful labels). This series of four blocks was presented twice, so the whole test consisted of eight blocks. Instructions were identical to those of the previous experiments. GY was not informed about the non-congruence between the stimuli and the labels he was instructed to use.

ERP recording and processing: Visual event-related brain potentials were recorded on two separate occasions using a Neuroscan with 64 channels. GY was tested in a dimly lit, electrically shielded room with the head restrained by a chin rest 60 cm from the screen, fixating a central cross. Four blocks of 240 stimuli were presented. Stimuli consisted of complex gray-scale and coloured static normal front faces taken from the Ekman series [14]. Three types of facial expressions appearing randomly either in the good visual field or in the blind visual field were presented (neutral, happy and fearful), for a total of 48 experimental conditions (2 visual hemi-fields × 2 colours × 3 emotions × 2 genders × 2 identities) each repeated 20 times. Stimulus duration was 1250 ms and the inter-trial interval was randomized between 1000 and 1500 ms. Stimuli were presented with the internal edge of the stimulus at 4.76 of the fixation cross in the center of the screen. Size of stimulus was 6 × 10 cm. Mean luminance of the room was <1 cd/m², 25 cd/m² for the face and <1 cd/m² for the screen in between stimulus presentations. When presented in his blind or good visual fields, GY was instructed to discriminate (or guess in the blind field) the gender of the faces by pressing one of two keys.

Horizontal EOG and vertical EOG were monitored using facial bipolar electrodes. EEG was recorded with a left ear reference and amplified with a gain of 30 K and band-pass filtered at 0.01–100 Hz. Impedance was kept below 5 kΩ. EEG and EOG were continuously acquired at a rate of 500 Hz. Epoching was performed 100 ms prior to stimulus onset and continued for 924 ms after stimulus presentation. Data were re-referenced off-line to a common average reference and low-pass filtered at 30 Hz. Amplitudes and latencies of visual components were measured relative to a 100 ms pre-stimulus baseline.

Results

Experiment 1:   Our first study used a total of 8 blocks consisting of different stimulus pairs (happy/sad, angry/sad, angry/fearful). The task was a 2AFC and GY was instructed to guess the facial expression shown to his blind field. GY was always flawless with stimuli presented to his intact left hemifield (LVF). When asked to report verbally what he saw in his damaged right hemifield (RVF), GY frequently reported detecting the offset and onset of a white flash, but he never consciously perceived a face or even a moving stimulus. Overall, 333 trials were presented in his right (blind) visual field (Table 1), and he was correct on 220 of them (66%, $Z = 5.86$, $p < 0.005$).

Experiment 2:   The second experiment used four different video fragments (happy/ sad/angry/fearful) presented in a four-alternative forced-choice design and shown

Table 1 Covert recognition of facial expressions

Stimulating pair	Image size	L/R presentation	Correct	p
Happy/fearful	Small	Randomized	22/27	<0.001
Happy/fearful	Large	Randomized	18/28	NS
Happy/fearful	Small	Blocked	37/58	<0.05
Happy/fearful	Large	Blocked	37/58	<0.05
Angry/sad	Small	Randomized	15/27	NS
Angry/sad	Small	Blocked	39/54	<0.01
Angry/fearful	Small	Randomized	15/27	NS
Angry/fearful	Small	Blocked	37/56	<0.05

Table 2 Confusion matrix of GYs response to happy, sad, angry, or fearful videos

Video	Response			
	Happy	Sad	Angry	Fearful
Happy	27	2	6	1
Sad	1	24	5	6
Angry	3	11	13	9
Fearful	2	12	6	15

in the RVF. GY correctly labeled the videos as happy, sad, angry, or fearful on 38 of 72 trials in the first block (52%, with the chance level at 25%; $Z = 5.30$, $p < 0.005$) and in 41 of 72 trials in the second block (57%; $Z = 6.12$, $p < 0.005$; Table 2). The happy and sad videos were recognized, as before, better than the angry and fearful videos. The overall performance was far above chance ($Z = 8.17$, $p < 0.005$). GY thus also performed well in a complex design that required more than a simple binary decision.

Experiment 3: The third experiment was carried out to assess whether movement was an important parameter for GY's performance or whether he can recognize stationary face expressions (stills). We used a 2AFC task and GY was instructed to guess the facial expression shown to his blind field. Per-formance with the video fragments was compared with those for still shots and for upside-down presentation. Table 3 shows that performance was better with moving stimuli than with still ones. Movement seems therefore to play an important role for GY in distinguishing facial expressions. This issue is further examined in the next experiment using congruent *vs* non-congruent labels, where movement was present throughout all presentations.

Experiment 4: To test whether performance was critically dependent on the veridical response labels being used, GY was tested a few months after Experiments 1–3. In the congruent blocks, GY had to identify the happy/sad videos with the labels happy/sad, or to identify the angry/fearful videos with the labels angry/fearful. In the non-congruent blocks, he was given the response labels angry or fearful, while, unknown to him, the happy/sad videos were presented, or conversely, he was given the labels happy/sad, while the angry/fearful videos were shown.

Table 3 Perceiving facial expressions or discriminating movement

Stimulus	Orientation	Presentation	Correct	p
Dynamic	Upright	Randomized	20/28	<0.05
Still	Upright	Randomized	19/27	<0.05
Dynamic	Inverted	Randomized	18/28	NS
Still	Inverted	Randomized	16/28	NS
Dynamic	Upright	Blocked	51/56	<0.001
Still	Upright	Blocked	26/53	NS
Dynamic	Inverted	Blocked	26/56	NS
Still	Inverted	Blocked	27/54	NS

GY did not report experiencing anything strange or different between congruent and non-congruent blocks. As before, he reported to detecting a white flash with an onset and an offset, but nothing more than that. However, performance was better with congruent labels.

In the first block, with congruent happy/sad videos and labels, GY was correct on 46 of 56 trials (four trials discarded for the presence of eye movements): 21 of 28 happy faces were recognized as happy, and 25 of 28 sad faces were recognized as sad ($\chi^2(1) = 23.62$, $p < 0.001$). On second testing, he was correct on 47 of 60 trials: 24 of 30 happy faces were recognized as happy, and 23 of 30 sad faces were recognized as sad ($\chi^2(1) = 19.28$, $p < 0.001$).

On the first test with congruent angry/fearful videos and labels, GY was correct on only 26 of 60 trials: 15 of 30 angry faces were recognized as angry, and 11 of 30 fearful faces were recognized as fearful ($\chi^2(1) = 1.08$, NS). On the second test, however, he improved considerably, and was correct on 40 of 60 trials: 21 of 30 angry faces were recognized as angry, and 19 of 30 fearful faces were recognized as fearful ($\chi^2(1) = 6.69$, $p < 0.01$). It thus appeared that the angry/fearful videos were more difficult than the happy/sad videos, but his performance improved on second time testing. Overall, GY was correct on 159/236 trials (67%; $\chi^2(1) = 28.51$, $p < 0.001$).

When presented with non-congruent angry/fearful videos and happy/sad labels (Table 4, top half) there was a clear majority of sad responses but without any relation

Table 4 GY's labeling of the videos with congruent and incongruent labels

Video	Response	
Angry/fearful videos		
	Happy	Sad
Angry	24	36
Fearful	24	36
Happy/sad videos		
	Fear	Angry
Happy	33	27
Sad	32	28

with the video that was shown ($\chi^2(1) = 0.00$, NS). The majority of sad responses presumably comes from an association of the negative emotion in both angry and fearful videos with the sad label. Using the non-congruent happy/sad videos and angry/fearful labels (Table 4, bottom half) the relative frequencies of the two response labels show very little relation to the presented videos ($\chi^2(1) = 1.11$, NS). With non-congruent labels, there was thus no systematic link between choice of response labels and the presented stimuli.

Event related brain potentials to facial expressions: The subject gave 92.8% correct responses in the good visual field and 51.4% in the blind visual field when discriminating the gender of static faces. This latter result is compatible with his difficulty in discriminating static faces in his blind field (see above).

Figure 1 shows grand-average visual ERPs for happy and fearful faces together at Oz site for left visual field presentation and right visual field presentations. Visual

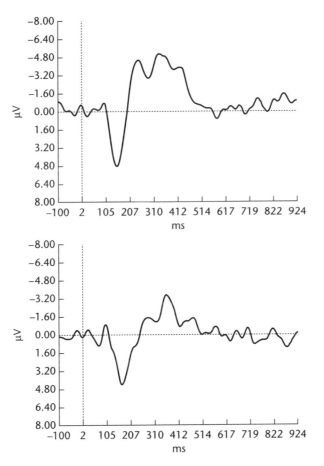

Figure 1 Grand-average visual ebvent-related potentials (VERPs) at Oz site for happy and fearful faces together. The upper part of the figure shows VERPs for presentations in the good visual hemifield, the lower part for presentations in the blind visual hemifield.

stimulations in the normal visual hemifield gave a first positive deflection peaking at 148.62 ms (amplitude 4.83 µV), followed by a subsequent negative visual component (latency 240.02 ms; amplitude −4.50 µV). Visual stimulations in the blind visual hemifield yielded a similar occipital positive component, delayed in time (164.04 ms) and slightly reduced in amplitude (4.44 µV). Moreover, a subsequent negative component was also seen (latency 276 ms; amplitude −1.50 µV) when GY was stimulated with faces in the blind visual hemifield.

The present electrophysiological data clearly show that early visually evoked activity can be found in ventro-lateral extrastriate cortex when stimuli are presented to the blind hemifield of a hemianopic subject. The first positive activity is entirely compatible (by latency and topography) with the P1 component generated in lateral extrastriate areas, near the border of Brodman areas 18 and 19 [15–17]. The second negative activity is compatible with a N1 component generated in the occipito-parietal and occipito-temporal cortex [16]. It has been suggested that the P1 component reflects processing in the ventral stream and that the N1 component processing in the dorsal stream [19]. Although reduced and delayed, neuronal activity elicited by stimulation of the blind visual hemifield is entirely comparable with face-related activity elicited by stimulation of the good visual hemifield.

Discussion

We have shown that a blindsight subject could discriminate successfully among different facial expressions and that this performance reflected actually a covert recognition of the facial expressions rather than a discrimination of two patterns of movement. Moreover, the actual conscious content of the alternative response labels he was given were particulary important for his performance since the subject performed better with congruent labels than with incongruent ones when the movement factor was kept constant. These observations are further supported by the electrophysiological results demonstrating that GY may activate the ventral visual pathway bypassing V1. An early visual activity is elicited in response to stimulation in the blind hemifield, and this activity is comparable and symmetric to the activity elicited in the other hemisphere in response to stimulations in the good visual hemifield. A delayed and reduced P1 and N1 components are indeed elicited at occipital sites (e.g. electrode Oz) in the left hemisphere in GY. The P1 component has been shown to be generated in extrastriate occipital regions but with a significant striate contribution as well [17]. The presence of a P1 component delayed in time and reduced in amplitude when GY was stimulated in his blind visual hemifield may be viewed as reflecting the absence of contribution of the left striate cortex lesioned in GY which should normally be involved in generating this early visual component in normal subjects [16,17]. Without further research it cannot be concluded just which specific features of the facial stimuli were critical for generating the pattern of ERPs recorded here, but the results show that such stimuli presented in the blind visual hemifield of an hemianopic subject activate the ventral visual pathway via anatomical routes that bypass V1. Connections from the retina to extrastriate areas via the pulvinar or the collicular-pulvinar pathway may yield such an early activity [4,18].

Conclusion

This study is the first to show processing of facial expressions in the absence of aware-ness in a subject with striate cortex lesion. Our report provides empirical evidences for the conjectures recently made by Morris *et al.* [4], suggesting a possible visual pathway bypassing V1 and involving the superior colliculus and the pulvinar which remain functional in a blindsight patient.

References

1. Morris, J.S., Friston, K.J., Büchel, C. *et al. Brain* **121**, 47–57 (1998).
2. Breiter, H.C., Etcoff, N.L., Whalen, P.J. *et al. Neuron* **17**, 875–887 (1996).
3. Whalen, P.J., Rauch, S.L., Etcoff, N.L. *et al. J Neurosci* **18**, 411–418 (1998).
4. Morris, J.S., Öhman, A. and Dolan, R.J. *Proc Natl Acad Sci USA* **96**, 1680–1685 (1999).
5. de Gelder, B., Pourtois, G., Vroomen, J. *et al.* Covert processing of facial expres-sions in prosopagnosia: Evidence from cross-modal bias. *Brain and Cognition* (in press).
6. Weiskrantz, L. *Blindsight: A Case Study and Implications.* Oxford: Oxford University Press, 1986.
7. Sahraie, A., Weiskrantz, L. and Barbur, J.L. *Behav Brain Res* **96**, 71–77 (1998).
8. Stoerig, P. and Cowey, A. *Nature* **342**, 916–918 (1989).
9. Stoerig, P. and Cowey, A. *Brain* **115**, 425–444 (1992).
10. Barbur, J.L., Sahraie, A., Simmons, A. *et al. Vis Res* **38**, 3347–3353 (1998).
11. Brent, P.J., Kennard, C. and Ruddock, K.H. *Proc R Soc Lond B Biol Sci* **256**, 219–225 (1994).
12. Marcel, A.J. *Brain* **121**, 1565–1588 (1998).
13. Weiskrantz, L. *et al. Brain* **121**, 1065–72 (1998).
14. Ekman, P. and Friesen, W.V. *J Environ Psychol Non-verbal Behav* **1**, 56–75 (1976).
15. Mangun, G.R. *Psychophysiology* **32**, 4–18 (1995).
16. Clark, V.P., Fan, S. and Hillyard, S.A. *Hum Brain Map* **2**, 170–187 (1995).
17. Martinez, A., Anllo-Vento, L., Sereno, M.I. *et al. Nature Neurosci* **2**, 364–369 (1999).
18. Mangun, G.R. and Hillyard, S.A. *Percept Psychophys* **47**, 532–550 (1990).
19. Stoerig, P. and Cowey, A. *Brain* **120**, 535–559 (1997).

ACKNOWLEDGEMENTS: This research was supported by ARC 95/00-189.
Received 18 August 1999; accepted 28 September 1999

Appendix 6 – Chapter 7

Navigation-related structural change in the hippocampi of taxi drivers

Maguire, E.A., Gadian, D.G., Johnsrude, I.S., Good, C.D., Ashburner, J., Frackowiak, R.S. and Frith, C.D. (2000)
Proceedings of the National Academy of Science, USA, 97(8): 4398–403.

Structural MRIs of the brains of humans with extensive navigation experience, licensed London taxi drivers, were analyzed and compared with those of control subjects who did not drive taxis. The posterior hippocampi of taxi drivers were significantly larger relative to those of control subjects. A more anterior hippocampal region was larger in control subjects than in taxi drivers. Hippocampal volume correlated with the amount of time spent as a taxi driver (positively in the posterior and negatively in the anterior hippocampus). These data are in accordance with the idea that the posterior hippocampus stores a spatial representation of the environment and can expand regionally to accommodate elaboration of this representation in people with a high dependence on navigational skills. It seems that there is a capacity for local plastic change in the structure of the healthy adult human brain in response to environmental demands.

One important role of the hippocampus is to facilitate spatial memory in the form of navigation (1). Increased hippocampal volume relative to brain and body size has been reported in small mammals and birds who engage in behavior requiring spatial memory, such as food storing (2). In some species, hippocampal volumes enlarge specifically during seasons when demand for spatial ability is greatest (2, 3). In the healthy human, structural brain differences between distinct groups of subjects (for example, males and females, ref. 4, or musicians and nonmusicians, ref. 5) have been documented. From existing studies, it is impossible to know whether differences in brain anatomy are predetermined or whether the brain is susceptible to plastic change in response to environmental stimulation. Furthermore, although lesion work (6, 7) and functional neuroimaging work (8) confirm the involvement of the human hippocampus in spatial memory and navigation, there is still debate about its precise role. Given the propensity of lower mammalian/avian hippocampi to undergo structural change in response to behavior requiring spatial memory (2, 3), the present study addressed whether morphological changes could be detected in the healthy human brain associated with extensive experience of spatial navigation. Our prediction was that the hippocampus would be the most likely brain region to show changes.

Taxi drivers in London must undergo extensive training, learning how to navigate between thousands of places in the city. This training is colloquially known as 'being on The Knowledge' and takes about 2 years to acquire on average. To be licensed to operate, it is necessary to pass a very stringent set of police examinations. London taxi drivers are therefore ideally suited for the study of spatial navigation. The use of a group of taxi drivers with a wide range of navigating experience permitted an examination of the direct effect of spatial experience on brain structure. In the first instance, we used voxel-based morphometry (VBM) to examine whether morphological changes associated with navigation experience were detectable anywhere in the healthy human brain. VBM is an objective and automatic procedure that identifies regional differences in relative gray matter density in structural MRI brain scans. It allows every point in the brain to be considered in an unbiased way, with no *a priori* regions of interest. The data were also analyzed by using a second and completely independent pixel-counting technique within the hippocampus proper. Comparisons were made between the brain scans of taxi drivers, who had all acquired a significant amount of large-scale spatial information (as evidenced by passing the licensing examinations), and those of a comparable group of control subjects who lacked such extensive navigation exposure.

Methods

Subjects. Right-handed male licensed London taxi drivers ($n = 16$; mean age 44 years; range 32–62 years) participated. All had been licensed London taxi drivers for more than 1.5 years (mean time as taxi driver = 14.3 years; range = 1.5–42 years). The average time spent training to be a taxi driver before passing the licensing tests fully (i.e., time on The Knowledge) was 2 years (range 10 months to 3.5 years; some trained continuously, some part time). All of the taxi drivers had healthy general medical, neurological, and psychiatric profiles. The scans of control subjects were selected from the structural MRI scan database at the same unit where the taxi drivers were scanned. Those subjects below 32 and above 62 years of age were excluded as were females, left-handed males, and those with any health problems. After the application of these exclusion criteria, the scans of 50 healthy right-handed males who did not drive taxis were included in the analyses for comparison with the taxi drivers. Both the mean age and the age range did not differ between the taxi driver and control groups. We were also careful to ensure an even spread of subjects in each decade (for example, 41–50 years or 51–60 years) up to the upper limit of the oldest taxi driver, such that subjects were not clustered at one end of the age scale.

Image Acquisition. Structural MRI scans were obtained with a 2.0 Tesla Vision system (Siemens GmbH, Erlangen, Germany) by using a T1-weighted three-dimensional gradient echo sequence (TR 9.7 ms; TE 4 ms; flip angle 12°; field of view 256 mm; 108 partitions; partition thickness 1.5 mm; voxel size $1 \times 1 \times 1.5$ mm).

Image Analysis Method 1: VBM. Data were analyzed by using VBM implemented with Statistical Parametric Mapping (SPM99, Wellcome Department of Cognitive Neurology) executed in MATLAB (Mathworks, Sherborn, MA). Detailed descriptions of the technique are given elsewhere (9, 10). Briefly, the subjects' data were spatially normalized into stereotactic space (11) by registering each of the images to the same template image by minimizing the residual sums of squared differences between them.

The template was generated from the structural scans of 50 healthy males acquired in the same scanner used to collect the data for the current analysis (the scans of 13 of the control subjects used in the VBM analysis were included in the creation of this template). The spatially normalized images were written in voxels of $1.5 \times 1.5 \times 1.5$ mm and segmented into gray matter, white matter, and cerebrospinal fluid by using a modified mixture cluster analysis technique. To reduce confounds caused by individual differences in gyral anatomy, the gray matter images were smoothed by using an isotropic Gaussian kernel of 4-mm full width at half maximum. The statistical model included a measure of total amount of gray matter in each brain as a confound (essentially the original values before normalization). Statistical tests involved locating regionally specific differences in gray matter between subject groups and were based on t tests and the general linear model. Significance levels were set at $P < 0.05$ (small volume correction for multiple comparisons, with 62 resolution elements comprising the volume of interest). To be consistent across the two analysis techniques, we defined the hippocampal regions the same way in both cases as described below.

Image Analysis Method 2: Pixel Counting. The three-dimensional images from the 16 taxi drivers and a precisely age-matched sample of 16 normal controls taken from the 50 used in the VBM analysis were submitted for region-of-interest-based volumetric measurement of both hippocampi by using a well established pixel-counting technique (12, 13). The images were analyzed by one person experienced in the technique and blinded to subjects' identity as taxi drivers or controls and the VBM findings. Briefly, the images were reformatted into 1.5-mm-thick contiguous sections in a tilted coronal plane that was perpendicular to the long axis of the hippocampus. Hippocampal cross-sectional areas were measured for each slice along the whole length of the hippocampus. There were at least 26 contiguous slices (each 1.5-mm-thick) for each hippocampus of each subject, giving a total length of approximately 4 cm. Total hippocampal volume was calculated by summing the cross-sectional areas and multiplying by the distance between adjacent slices (i.e., 1.5 mm). These volumes were then corrected for intracranial volume (ICV), which was measured from the sagittal slices of the original three-dimensional data sets. Measurements for the most posterior slices violated assumptions of homogeneity of variance and were therefore not considered in the analyses, leaving the measurements for 24 slices. These were grouped into three regions (14): posterior hippocampus (6 slices), body (12 slices), and anterior (6 slices). Values for the component slices for a particular region were averaged, and the data were analyzed by ANOVA and correlations (significance level set at $P < 0.05$). We report the analyses on data uncorrected for ICV (when data were corrected for ICV, the results did not differ).

Results

VBM. Significantly increased gray matter volume was found in the brains of taxi drivers compared with those of controls in only two brain regions, namely the right and the left hippocampi (Figure 1a and b). No differences were observed elsewhere in the brain. The increase in hippocampal gray matter volume was focal and limited to

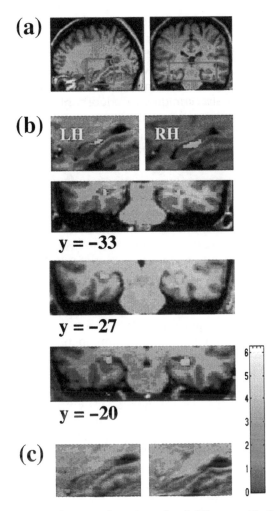

Figure 1 VBM findings. (*a Left*) Sagittal section of an MRI scan with the hippocampus indicated by the red box. (*a Right*) Coronal section through the MRI scan, again with the hippocampi indicated. (*b*) The group results are shown superimposed onto the scan of an individual subject selected at random. The bar to the right indicates the *Z* score level. Increased gray matter volume in the posterior of the left and right hippocampi (LH and RH, respectively) of taxi drivers relative to those of controls, shown in the top of the figure in sagittal section. Underneath, the areas of gray matter difference are shown in coronal sections at three different coordinates in the *y* axis to illustrate the extent of the difference down the long axis of the hippocampus. (*c*) Increased gray matter volume in the anterior of the left and right hippocampi of controls relative to those of taxi drivers, shown in sagittal section. Note that, although the Talairach and Tournoux (11) coordinate system was used to describe the locations of VBM differences in stereotactic space, the images were normalized with respect to a template based on a large number of brains scanned in the same scanner used to collect the current data (see *Methods*). Thus, the coordinates given refer to our brain template and only approximately to the Talairach and Tournoux template.

the posterior hippocampus bilaterally. The voxel of peak difference in gray matter density in the right hippocampus was at (x, y, z) 31, −22, −13 ($Z = 4.34$) and, in the left hippocampus, was at −31, −28, −10 ($Z = 4.19$). The area of difference extended in the y axis in the right hippocampus from −17 mm to −33 mm and in the left hippocampus from −18 mm to −34 mm. Controls showed a relatively greater gray matter volume bilaterally in anterior hippocampi relative to those of taxi drivers (Figure 1c). The voxel of peak difference in gray matter density in the right hippocampus was at 32, −7, −28 ($Z = 2.65$) and in the left hippocampus was at −34, −7, −26 ($Z = 2.65$). The anterior changes did not survive correction for multiple comparisons but were confirmed in the second analysis technique as described below.

Pixel Counting. Hippocampal volumes (both corrected and uncorrected for ICV) and ICV did not differ significantly between the two subject groups [right hippocampus: taxi drivers, uncorrected = 4,300 mm³ (± 432), corrected = 4,159 mm³ (± 420); controls, uncorrected = 4,255 mm³ (± 424), corrected = 4,080 mm³ (± 325); left hippocampus: taxi drivers, uncorrected = 4,155 mm³ (± 410), corrected = 3,977 mm³ (± 350); controls, uncorrected = 4,092 mm³ (± 324), corrected = 3,918 mm³ (± 224); ICV of taxi drivers = 1,521 mm³ (± 145); controls = 1,540 mm³ (± 107)].

Although the analysis revealed no difference in the overall volume of the hippocampi between taxi drivers and controls, it did reveal regionally specific differences in volume (Figure 2). ANOVA (group by side) on anterior hippocampal volumes revealed a main effect of group, with control volumes significantly greater than those in taxi drivers [df (1, 30); $F = 5$; $P < 0.05$], a main effect of side, with the anterior right hippocampus being larger than the left [df (1, 30); $F = 4.5$; $P < 0.05$], and no interaction. Analysis of the volumes for the body of the hippocampus showed no interaction and no effect of group but a main effect of side, again right greater than left [df (1, 30); $F = 5.4$; $P < 0.05$]. Finally, analysis of volumes of the posterior hippocampus revealed a main effect of group, with taxi drivers having a greater posterior hippocampal volume than controls [df (1, 30); $F = 4.1$; $P < 0.05$]. Neither the interaction nor the main effect of side was significant.

Changes with Navigation Experience. We examined the correlation between volume and amount of time spent as a taxi driver (including both training on The Knowledge and practicing as a qualified taxi driver). We found that length of time spent as a taxi driver correlated positively with volume in only one brain region, the right posterior hippocampus (Figure 3a). Correction for age was made by including it as a confounding covariate. The voxel of peak correlation in the right hippocampus was at 22, −33, 3 ($Z = 5.65$). The extent of the area in the right hippocampus ranged in the y axis from −29 mm to −36 mm. The spatial extent of this area overlapped with the area showing greater volume in the categorical comparison of taxi drivers with controls. The VBM changes as a function of time (in months) spent as a taxi driver (corrected for age effects) and global gray matter are plotted in Figure 3b, where the data were considered within a linear model ($r = 0.6$; $P < 0.05$). The correlation between time spent as a taxi driver (corrected for age) and the pixel-counting data indicated a similar relationship for the posterior hippocampus ($r = 0.5$; $P < 0.06$). The pixel-counting data also showed a negative correlation between the time spent as a taxi driver and the

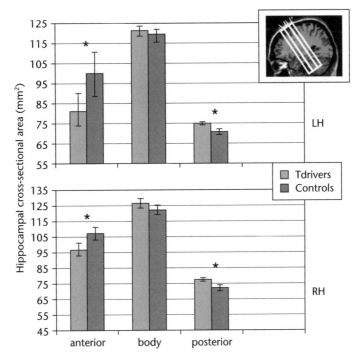

Figure 2 Volumetric analysis findings. The orientation of the slices measured in the volumetric analysis with respect to the hippocampus is shown (*Top Right Inset*). A, anterior; B, body; P, posterior. (*Upper*) The mean of the cross-sectional area measurements (uncorrected for ICV) for the three regions of the left hippocampus (LH). (*Lower*) The means for the right hippocampus (RH). Taxi drivers had a significantly greater volume relative to controls in the posterior hippocampus, and controls showed greater hippocampal volume in the anterior. There was no difference between the two groups in the hippocampus body. *, $P < 0.05$.

volume of anterior hippocampal tissue ($r = -0.6$; $P < 0.05$) as plotted in Figure 3c. When time as a taxi driver was corrected for age by expressing it as a percentage of age, the result was identical ($r = -0.6$; $P < 0.05$). The data of one taxi driver were not included in the correlation analyses. He had been a taxi driver for 42 years, and the next nearest length of time was 28 years; thus, he was treated as an outlier and removed. The data of this subject were completely in line with the relationships as plotted; for example, his VBM response measure was 13.7.

Discussion

The data presented in this report provide evidence of regionally specific structural differences between the hippocampi of licensed London taxi drivers compared with those of control subjects. Taxi drivers had a significantly greater volume in the posterior hippocampus, whereas control subjects showed greater volume in the anterior

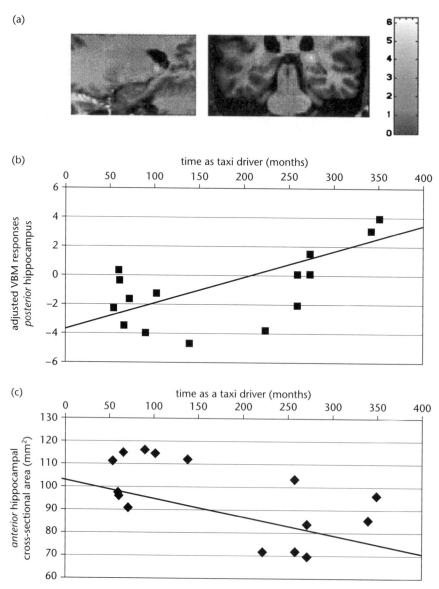

Figure 3 Correlation of volume change with time as a taxi driver. (*a Left*) Sagittal section. (*a Right*) Coronal section. The VBM group results are shown superimposed onto the scan of an individual subject selected at random. The bar to the right indicates the *Z* score level. The volume of gray matter in the right hippocampus was found to correlate significantly with the amount of time spent learning to be and practicing as a licensed London taxi driver, positively in the right posterior hippocampus (*b*) and negatively in the anterior hippocampus (*c*).

hippocampus. The converging results from these two independent analysis techniques indicate that the professional dependence on navigational skills in licensed London taxi drivers is associated with a relative redistribution of gray matter in the hippocampus. We further considered whether the volume differences between the groups could be incidental and unassociated with the navigational requirements of the taxi drivers. For example, could this particular arrangement of hippocampal gray matter predispose individuals to professional dependence on navigational skills? Although this explanation would be fascinating in itself, we tested this notion directly by examining the correlation between volume and amount of time spent as a taxi driver. Right hippocampal volume correlated with the amount of time spent as a taxi driver (positively in the posterior and negatively in the anterior hippocampus). We believe that these data suggest that the changes in hippocampal gray matter – at least on the right – are acquired. As such, this finding indicates the possibility of local plasticity in the structure of the healthy adult human brain as a function of increasing exposure to an environmental stimulus.

Previous rodent and monkey studies have found the dorsal (posterior) hippocampus to be preferentially involved in spatial navigation (15–18). Such an involvement may also be true for the rostral part of the hippocampus in birds (19). There are also many more cells with spatial correlates – place cells (20) – in the dorsal than in the ventral rat hippocampus (21). Functional neuroimaging studies of navigation in humans show that the retrieval or use of previously learned navigational information is associated with activation of the posterior hippocampus (22–24). Patients with lesions of the hippocampus that spare the posterior aspect have been reported to be unimpaired at recalling routes learned before lesion onset (6). Exactly how much posterior hippocampus needs to be spared to support the recall of 'old' cognitive maps is not clear. For instance, it has been reported recently that a patient with extensive damage to the medial temporal region bilaterally, including the hippocampus, could recall the town where he grew up many years before (25). The authors of that report inferred from this fact that the medial temporal region is not the repository of spatial maps. However, they also allude to some sparing of the hippocampal tissue near the lateral ventricles bilaterally. It is therefore not clear whether this tissue was contributing to the recall of the patient's spatial map. Unfortunately, the patient was not tested by using functional neuroimaging during the recall of these old memories, which could have confirmed whether the remaining hippocampal tissue was still functional. We would predict that it was.

Our finding that the posterior hippocampus increases in volume when there is occupational dependence on spatial navigation is evidence for functional differentiation within the hippocampus. In humans, as in other animals, the posterior hippocampus seems to be preferentially involved when previously learned spatial information is used, whereas the anterior hippocampal region may be more involved (in combination with the posterior hippocampus) during the encoding of new environmental layouts.

A basic spatial representation of London is established in the taxi drivers by the time The Knowledge is complete. This representation of the city is much more extensive in taxi drivers than in the control subjects. Among the taxi drivers, there is, over time and with experience, a further fine-tuning of the spatial representation of London, permitting increasing understanding of how routes and places relate to each other.

Our results suggest that the 'mental map' of the city is stored in the posterior hippocampus and is accommodated by an increase in tissue volume. These results challenge the traditional view that the hippocampus has a transient role in memory (26) at least in relation to spatial navigation and the posterior hippocampus. The need to navigate is a basic cross-species behavior. The hippocampus is a phylogenetically old part of the brain, with an intrinsic circuitry that may have evolved to deal with navigation. Undoubtedly, in humans, the functions of the hippocampus have adapted to accommodate other types of memory, such as episodic memory (27–29), but the hippocampus retains an ability to store large-scale spatial information (1).

Our findings from two independent measurement techniques are consistent with patient (6) and functional neuroimaging (22) reports of bilateral hippocampal involvement in successful navigation. Unlike right hippocampal volume, however, left hippocampal volume did not correlate with years of taxi-driving experience, suggesting that the left hippocampus participates in spatial navigation and memory in a different way from the right hippocampus. We may speculate that the left hippocampus complements its partner by storing memories of people and events that occur in the rich context of taxi driving in the real world, where an over-arching framework – such as integrating information into an existing map – is not required (30).

Although the hippocampus does not support navigation in isolation from other brain regions, it seems to be crucial to the storage and use of mental maps of our environments. The prolonged accumulation of other types of nonnavigational information may also produce similar hippocampal changes. Our present findings, however, corroborated as they are by the results of patient and neuroimaging studies, suggest that space and the posterior right human hippocampus are intimately linked.

Given the macroscopic level of our analyses, the data do not speak directly to the microscopic mechanisms, such as neurogenesis (31–33), that might underlie the structural change we report herein. The differential changes in posterior and anterior hippocampus may represent two separate processes. The most parsimonious explanation, however, is that our findings reflect an overall internal reorganization of hippocampal circuitry (34) in response to a need to store an increasingly detailed spatial representation, where changes in one hippocampal region are very likely to affect others. On a broader level, the demonstration that normal activities can induce changes in the relative volume of gray matter in the brain has obvious implications for rehabilitation of those who have suffered brain injury or disease. It remains to be seen whether similar environment-related plasticity is possible in other regions of the human brain outside of the hippocampus.

E.A.M., I.S.J., C.D.G., J.A., R.S.J.F., and C.D.F. are supported by the Wellcome Trust. D.G.G. thanks the Wellcome Trust for its support at the Institute of Child Health. We are grateful for the assistance of Helen Gallagher, Amanda Brennan, and Jon Galliers. We also thank Andrew Holmes, Cheryl Johnson, and David McGonigle.

Note

Abbreviations: VBM, voxel-based morphometry; ICV, intracranial volume.

References

1. O'Keefe, J. and Nadel, L. (1978) *The Hippocampus as a Cognitive Map* (Clarendon, Oxford).
2. Lee, D.W., Miyasato, L.E. and Clayton, N.S. (1998) *NeuroReport* **9**, R15–R27.
3. Smulders, T.V., Sasson, A.D. and DeVoogd, T.J. (1995) *J. Neurobiol.* **27**, 15–25.
4. Gur, R.C., Turetsky, B.I., Matsui, M., Yan, M., Bilker, W., Hughett, P. and Gur, R.E. (1999) *J. Neurosci.* **19**, 4065–4072.
5. Schlaug, G., Jancke, L., Huang, Y. and Steinmetz, H. (1995) *Science* **267**, 699–701.
6. Maguire, E.A., Burke, T., Phillips, J. and Staunton, H. (1996) *Neuropsychologia* **34**, 993–1001.
7. Smith, M.L. and Milner, B. (1981) *Neuropsychologia* **19**, 781–793.
8. Maguire, E.A., Burgess, N. and O'Keefe, J. (1999) *Curr. Opin. Neurobiol.* **9**, 171–177.
9. Wright, I.C., McGuire, P.K., Poline, J.-B., Travere, J.M., Murray, R.M., Frith, C.D., Frackowiak, R.S.J. and Friston, K.J. (1995) *Neuroimage* **2**, 244–252.
10. May, A., Ashburner, J., Büchel, C., McGonigle, D.J., Friston, K.J., Frackowiak, R.S.J. and Goadsby, P.J. (1999) *Nat. Med.* **5**, 836–838.
11. Talairach, J. and Tournoux, P. (1988) *Coplanar Stereotactic Atlas of the Human Brain* (Thieme, Stuttgart).
12. Van Paesschen, W., Connolly, A., King, M.D., Jackson, G.D. and Duncan, J.S. (1997) *Ann. Neurol.* **41**, 41–51.
13. Vargha-Khadem, F., Gadian, D.G., Watkins, K.E., Connelly, A., Van Paesschen, W. and Mishkin, M. (1997) *Science* **277**, 376–380.
14. Duvernoy, H.M. (1998) *The Human Hippocampus* (Springer, Berlin).
15. Moser, M.B., Moser, E.I., Forrest, E., Andersen, P. and Morris, R.G. (1995) *Proc. Natl. Acad. Sci. USA* **92**, 9697–9701.
16. Moser, E.I., Moser, M.B. and Andersen, P. (1993) *J. Neurosci.* **13**, 3916–3925.
17. Hock, B.J. and Bunsey, M.D. (1998) *J. Neurosci.* **18**, 7027–7032.
18. Colombo, M., Fernandez, T., Nakamura, K. and Gross, C.G. (1998) *J. Neurophysiol.* **80**, 1002–1005.
19. Clayton, N.S. (1995) *Hippocampus* **5**, 499–510.
20. O'Keefe, J. and Dostrovsky, J. (1971) *Brain Res.* **34**, 171–175.
21. Jung, M.W., Wiener, S.I. and McNaughton, B.L. (1994) *J. Neurosci.* **14**, 7347–7356.
22. Maguire, E.A., Burgess, N., Donnett, J.G., Frackowiak, R.S.J., Frith, C.D. and O'Keefe, J. (1998) *Science* **280**, 921–924.
23. Maguire, E.A., Frackowiak, R.S.J. and Frith, C.D. (1997) *J. Neurosci.* **17**, 7103–7110.
24. Ghaem, O., Mellet, E., Crivello, F., Tzourio, N., Mazoyer, B., Berthoz, A. and Denis, M. (1997) *NeuroReport* **8**, 739–744.
25. Teng, E. and Squire, L.R. (1999) *Nature (London)* **400**, 675–677.
26. Squire, L.R. and Knowlton, B. (1995) in *The Cognitive Neurosciences*, ed. Gazzaniga, M.S. (MIT Press, Cambridge, MA), pp. 825–837.
27. Tulving, E. and Markovitsch, H.J. (1998) *Hippocampus* **8**, 198–204.
28. Squire, L.R. and Zola, S.M. (1998) *Hippocampus* **8**, 205–211.
29. Mishkin, M., Vargha-Khadem, F. and Gadian, D.G. (1998) *Hippocampus* **8**, 212–216.
30. Maguire, E.A. and Mummery, C.J. (1999) *Hippocampus* **9**, 54–61.

31. Gould, E., Tanapat, P., Hastings, N.B. and Shors, T. (1999) *Trends Cognit. Sci.* **3**, 186–192.
32. Kempermann, G., Kuhn, H.G. and Gage, F.H. (1998) *J. Neurosci.* **18**, 3206–3212.
33. Gould, E., Reeves, A.J., Graziano, M.S.A. and Gross, C.G. (1999) *Science* **286**, 548–552.
34. Rapp, P.R., Stack, E.C. and Gallagher, M. (1999) *J. Comp. Neurol.* **403**, 459–470.

Appendix 7 – Chapter 8

Coming Unbound: Disrupting Automatic Integration of Synesthetic Color and Graphemes by Transcranial Magnetic Stimulation of the Right Parietal Lobe

Esterman, M., Verstynen, T., Ivry, R.B. and Robertson, L.C. (2006)
Journal of Cognitive Neuroscience, 18(9): 1570–6.

Abstract

In some individuals, a visually presented letter or number automatically evokes the perception of a specific color, an experience known as color–grapheme synesthesia. It has been suggested that parietal binding mechanisms play a role in the phenomenon. We used a noninvasive stimulation technique, transcranial magnetic stimulation (TMS), to determine whether the posterior parietal lobe is critical for the integration of color and shape in color–grapheme synesthesia, as it appears to be for normal color–shape binding. Using a color-naming task with colored letters that were either congruent or incongruent with the synesthetic photism, we demonstrate that inhibition of the right posterior parietal lobe with repetitive TMS transiently attenuates synesthetic binding. These findings suggest that synesthesia (the induction of color from shape) relies on similar mechanisms as found in normal perception (where the perception of color is induced by wavelength).

Introduction

In color–grapheme synesthesia, specific graphemes are automatically seen in specific colors. For example, the letter 'A' is always perceived in a particular shade of red. This unusual variety of color–form binding has been well characterized behaviorally. However, the neural correlates of synesthesia are not well understood (Rich & Mattingley, 2002). Although functional magnetic resonance imaging (fMRI) has shown that increased activity in extrastriate cortex is associated with the perception of synesthetic photisms (Sperling, Prvulovic, Linden, Singer, & Stirn, 2006; Hubbard, Arman, Ramachandran, & Boynton, 2005), other brain imaging studies of color–grapheme synesthesia have shown neural correlates outside of the ventral occipital cortex in the posterior parietal cortex (PPC). Rich et al. (2003) found activation in the right PPC (at the junction of the occipital cortex) during synesthetic color–grapheme perception, an area implicated in normal binding of color and shape (Donner et al.,

2002). Others have found activation in the intraparietal sulcus (IPS) associated with color–grapheme synesthesia, both in the left hemisphere (Weiss, Zilles, & Fink, 2005) and bilaterally (Elias, Saucier, Hardie, & Sarty, 2003).

The PPC has already been associated with color–form binding in normal perception using tasks that involve conjunction visual search (Donner et al., 2002; Ashbridge, Walsh, & Cowey, 1997). In addition, patients with bilateral PPC lesions have difficulty in correctly conjoining shape and color. For example, R.M., a patient with Balint's syndrome, makes frequent illusory conjunctions in free viewing conditions (Friedman-Hill, Robertson, & Treisman, 1995). Together, these findings suggest that although synesthesia is an atypical integration of color and shape, it may rely on similar mechanisms to normal perceptual feature binding (Cohen-Kadosh & Henik, 2006; Sagiv, Heer, & Robertson, 2006; Robertson, 2003; Grossenbacher & Lovelace, 2001).

Further evidence that parietal mechanisms may be involved in synesthesia come from behavioral studies demonstrating that binding of the synesthetic photism requires awareness of the inducing grapheme and is modulated by whether the grapheme is within the spotlight of attention (Sagiv et al., 2006; Palmeri, Blake, Marois, Flanery, & Whetsell, 2002; Mattingley, Rich, Yelland, & Bradshaw, 2001). The idea that synesthesia arises from operations of an attentional binding mechanism is challenged by findings indicating preattentive activation of synesthetic percepts (Smilek, Dixon, & Merikle, 2004; Ramachandran & Hubbard, 2001). These contradictory results may be explained in part by individual differences between synesthetes (Hubbard & Ramachandran, 2005).

We sought to test the hypothesis that parietal binding mechanisms that are necessary for normal perception also play a role in color–grapheme synesthesia. To this end, we used a color-naming task (Mattingley et al., 2001; Dixon, Smilek, Cudahy, & Merikle, 2000). On each trial, a colored letter was presented in one of three colors and the participant pressed a key to indicate the color. The color was either congruent or incongruent with the synesthetic photism (Figure 1B). Synesthetic facilitation occurs when responses to letters presented in their synesthetic color (congruent condition) are *faster* than baseline responses (neutral characters that do not evoke a synesthetic

(A)
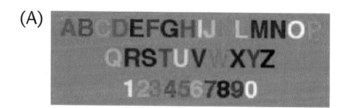

Figure 1 Behavioral and TMS procedure for participant E.F. (A) Synesthetic alphabet. (B) Individualized experimental conditions. The task was to name the stimulus color. In the congruent condition, the stimulus color matched the synesthetic color. In the incongruent condition, the stimulus color did not match the synesthetic color. Neutral characters did not evoke a synesthetic color. (C) Target stimulation site (right IPS/TOS) shown on coronal and axial slices, plus a 3-D reconstruction of the anatomical image for E.F. Target location is shown in red, center of magnetic coil is shown as green spheres in the 3-D image, and estimated pulse and orthogonal trajectories are shown as yellow lines.

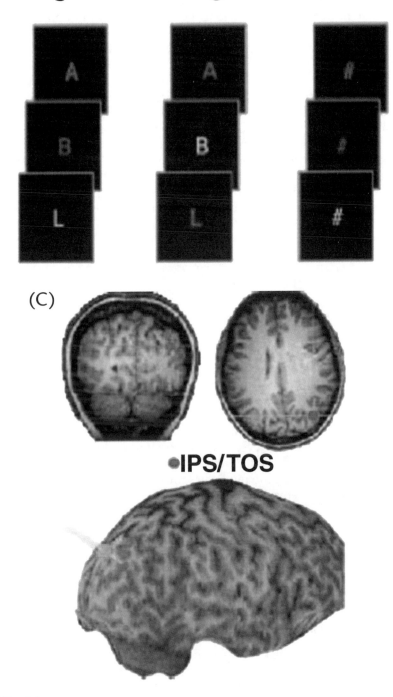

(B) Congruent   Incongruent   Neutral

(C)

●IPS/TOS

Figure 1 *(Cont'd)*

photism). Synesthetic interference occurs when responses to letters presented in colors that are incongruent with their synesthetic photism (incongruent condition) are *slower* than baseline. This task was performed following transcranial magnetic stimulation (TMS) of the left or right parietal cortex. This method allowed us to investigate whether transient inhibition of the parietal cortex influenced synesthetic induction of color by shape. Specifically, would parietal stimulation reduce any photism-induced facilitation or interference? Such changes would be consistent with this region contributing to binding of color and shape in synesthesia.

We targeted the angular gyrus at the junction of the posterior IPS and transverse occipital sulcus (IPS/TOS), a region associated with color–form binding in normal perception (Donner et al., 2002). In addition, activation in the right IPS/TOS has been observed during synesthetic color–grapheme perception (Rich et al., 2003), suggesting a correspondence between normal and synesthetic binding of color and form. In separate sessions, stimulation was applied over this parietal region of the right and left hemisphere. In another session, repetitive TMS (rTMS) was applied over the primary visual cortex (V1) to test for the effects of generalized brain stimulation on responses in this task.

Methods

Participants

All procedures for this experiment were approved by the local ethical review board at University of California at Berkeley. We tested two color–grapheme synesthetes recruited from the local population at the university: C.P. (27 years old) and E.F. (22 years old), both right-handed women. Both report having a unique set of alphanumeric–color associations (see Figure 1A) that are stable over time. Both reported their colors were projected in the external world and appeared as a 'property' of the inducing character, which was also in the 'mind's eye.' Both synesthetes would be classified as 'projectors' (Sagiv et al., 2006; Dixon, Smilek, & Merikle, 2004). It has been shown in a prior behavioral study that attention modulates the extent of C.P.'s synesthetic experience (Sagiv et al., 2006). Moreover, her experiences were previously associated with modest activation of lower visual areas, leading to her classification as a 'higher synesthete' (see participant C.H.P. in Hubbard et al., 2005).

We did not test participants with normal perception in this study because they have no synesthetic photism to influence color naming (see behavioral procedures described below) and training controls with color–grapheme associations would not replicate the experience of synesthesia.

Behavioral Procedure

Before testing, we estimated the specific RGB screen values for each letter of each participant's synesthetic alphabet. They were seated comfortably ~30 cm in front of a 19-in. CRT monitor (70 Hz refresh rate). An alphanumeric symbol was presented on the screen and the participant was instructed to adjust the RGB values until the color on the screen matched their synesthetic photism. For testing, we chose those letters that evoked the most red, green, and yellow color associations, respectively. Each shade of red, green, and yellow was chosen to closely match the synesthetic photism.

To quantify each participant's synesthesia we used a color-naming task. A series of colored single letters (red, green, or yellow; see above) were presented, each for 1000 msec, in a color that was either congruent (congruent trials) or incongruent (incongruent trials) with the synesthetic photism, or a symbol ('#') was presented that did not evoke a synesthetic photism (neutral trials; see Figure 1B for examples). Participants pressed a button with their right hand indicating the true color of the letter as quickly as possible while trying to ignore the synesthetic photism. Reaction time to manually respond to the screen color was recorded as the difference between the onset of the letter and the subsequent keypress. There was no deadline to respond. Following a response, there was a 1000 msec intertrial interval. Stimuli were presented with PsychLab software (Teren Gum, Boston, VA), and recorded with a CMU button box (three buttons pressed with three different fingers).

Each block consisted of 120 trials (48 congruent, 48 incongruent, and 24 neutral, representing all combinations of colors and characters). After each stimulation epoch (sham rTMS or real rTMS; see below), participants were tested on two blocks of trials: an early block (1–5 min poststimulation) and a late block (6–10 min poststimulation). Order of sham and real TMS was counterbalanced for each participant. Each sham and real TMS epoch was performed twice in each session, alternating between stimulation types. Separate sessions were done for each target region (right parietal, left parietal, V1). For each session, 960 trials were collected per participant.

Transcranial Magnetic Stimulation

We first obtained high-resolution anatomical MRIs for each participant. The images for C.P. were acquired in a previous study using a MPRAGE sequence on a 1.5T Siemens Vision scanner at the University of California, San Diego ($1 \times 1 \times 1$ isotropic voxels, 180 slices). The images for E.F. were acquired using a MPFLASH protocol on a Varian INNOVA 4T system at the University of California, Berkeley ($2 \times 2 \times 2$ isotropic voxels, 128 slices). We identified the target regions for TMS stimulation from each participant's MRI (left and right IPS/TOS and V1). The voxel location was marked on a skull-stripped reconstructed image.

The scalp location was determined by using a stereotaxic localization system (Brainsight, Rogue-Research Inc., Montreal, Canada). Coil position over the target regions was monitored online during the stimulation epochs. In addition, trajectory estimates of the TMS pulse were estimated intermittently throughout recording (green dots and yellow lines in Figure 1C). Although we chose our region of interest (ROI) based on each individual's anatomy, we estimated the Talairach coordinates of the right IPS/TOS site as (30, −74, 32), close to the area associated with feature binding (22, −71, 27) in Donner et al. (2002). Talairach space is primarily driven by the need to standardize across individuals and assumes a standard sulcal and gyral geometry. By nature, it is insensitive to individual differences in brain structure. The locations in the present study were identified by using the pattern of gross anatomical landmarks of the IPS, angular gyrus, and TOS. Thus, this coordinate is only an estimate of our stimulation location.

rTMS was performed by using an iron-cored figure-8 coil (NeoTonus Inc., Marietta, GA; see Epstein & Davey, 2002). Before each session, the participant's active motor threshold was determined as the point at which four to six visible twitches of the thumb were detected following 10 pulses over the motor cortex while the thumb and index finger were held together in a pinchlike posture. C.P.'s threshold was between 35 per cent and 38 per cent maximum stimulator output, whereas E.F.'s threshold was consistent at 45 per cent. Stimulation was then set to 115 per cent of motor threshold for the remainder of the experiment. Each stimulation epoch consisted of 480 consecutive pulses that were delivered at a rate of 1 Hz (8 min). This low-frequency design causes a transient inhibition of the underlying cortex, with the duration of the effect roughly equal to the duration of the stimulation at 1 Hz (Pascual-Leone et al., 1998). Thus, maximal behavioral effects of TMS were expected during the early block (minutes 1–5 post stimulation) diminishing during the late block (minutes 6–10 post stimulation). During rTMS blocks, the coil was oriented to deliver stimulation directly to the target cortical location. For sham control rTMS blocks, the coil was oriented 90° away from the scalp so that no pulses perturbed underlying neural tissue. The subjects were naive to whether they were receiving sham or real stimulation.

Data Analysis

Given the small sample size and the propensity for large between-subjects variability with synesthesia, we adopted a strong within-subject method to analyze the stimulation effects. The TMS effects were statistically analyzed by using randomization methods on a single-subject basis (e.g., bootstrapping; see Manly, 1997). All analyses excluded any reaction times greater than four standard deviations from the mean (less than 1 per cent of trials for each participant). We first recorded the interference effect for each of the six conditions (3 regions × 2 rTMS/sham epochs) by subtracting reaction times to incongruent trials from neutral trials. A 'true' TMS effect score (X_t) was determined by subtracting the interference effect observed following sham stimulation from the effect found after real rTMS. A score of zero indicates no change in interference following rTMS, a positive score indicates *increased* interference following rTMS, and a negative score represents a *decreased* interference effect after rTMS. We then randomly recategorized reaction times between neutral and incongruent trials and recalculated a new interference effect. This was done separately for rTMS and sham trials, following which a new TMS effect score was calculated. This scrambling, recategorization, and subtraction process was repeated for 10,000 iterations to produce a hypothetical probability distribution of interference effects that would occur simply by chance. Figure 2A shows an example of a random distribution of interference effects for C.P. following right-hemisphere stimulation. The dashed line represents her true TMS effect. These distributions closely resembled normal distributions, as verified using probability plots (Figure 2B; Chambers, Cleveland, Kleiner, & Tukey, 1983).

The probability of getting the true observed effects by chance (p) can then be directly calculated as:

$$p = \Sigma(X_r > X_t)$$

where X_r is the array of values pulled from the randomized null distribution.

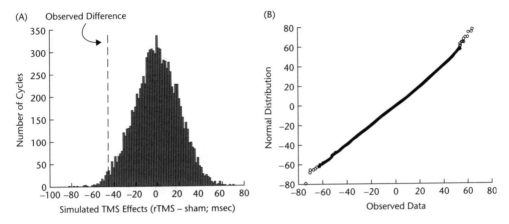

Figure 2 (A) A histogram of simulated TMS effects representing a hypothetical null distribution for C.P. after right PPC stimulation. The observed reaction times were randomly recategorized (with replacement) and new interference effects were calculated from these permutated data sets. This process was repeated 10,000 times to produce a distribution of values that represent what would be observed purely by chance. The dashed line represents the true observed TMS effect immediately following stimulation. (B) A normal probability plot, comparing the data presented in (A) with values from a normal distribution with mean of −0.04 msec and standard deviation of 20 msec. The approximately straight line indicates that the hypothetical null distribution reflect a normal gaussian process.

Results and discussion

Following sham rTMS, both participants showed synesthetic interference in all six blocks (E.F.: mean = 51 msec, range 32–90 msec; C.P.: mean = 31 msec; range, 19–48 msec). In contrast, rTMS of the right parietal ROI significantly attenuated interference for both participants during the early test block (by 54 msec for E.F. and 48 msec for C.P., $p < .01$; see Figure 3). For E.F., interference returned to baseline levels in the late block (61 msec); however, C.P.'s scores were still attenuated (10 msec), suggesting the effects of rTMS had not completely worn off. C.P.'s responses were generally faster overall following real rTMS, likely due to generalized arousal. More importantly, the attenuation of interference seen after right IPS/TOS stimulation is the result of a *disproportionate* decrease in reaction times on incongruent trials (see Table 1).

In contrast to right-hemisphere stimulation, rTMS over the left PPC had no effect on interference (see Figure 3; C.P.: $p = .22$, E.F.: $p = .09$). Thus, the disruption of synesthesia following right parietal rTMS does not generalize to the left-hemisphere homologue. This is consistent with neurophysiological evidence that the right parietal cortex plays a more critical role in normal color–form binding than does the left parietal cortex (Ashbridge et al., 1997).

rTMS over V1 also had no effect on interference (see Figure 3; C.P.: $p = .28$, E.F.: $p = .21$). Thus, the disruption of synesthesia following right parietal rTMS is not due to generalized arousal following stimulation and suggests that V1 does not play a critical role in color–form binding.

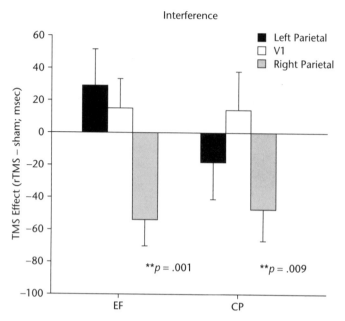

Figure 3 Effects of TMS on synesthetic interference. Graph displays effects of rTMS on synesthetic interference (incongruent minus neutral) for both participants immediately following stimulation (early block; see text). Both participants demonstrated a strong attenuation of interference following right parietal compared to sham rTMS, but no change following stimulation of the left parietal region or V1 (see Methods for discussion of statistical procedure and Table 1 for reaction times and standard deviations in all conditions).

Unlike interference, facilitation was not reliably observed in our participants. Naming colors that were synesthetically congruent produced consistently faster responses for participant E.F. only (36 msec). C.P. did not show consistent facilitation in the sham blocks (mean = 14 msec; range, −26 to 44 msec). Facilitation is not reliably observed in traditional Stroop tasks in normal observers (Tzelgov, Henik, & Berger, 1992; MacLeod, 1991) as well as tasks similar to ours when tested in other synesthetes (Sagiv et al., 2006; Mattingley et al., 2001; Dixon et al., 2000). It has been proposed that facilitation, when observed in traditional Stroop tasks, may be due to inadvertent reading, which would explain our weak facilitation effect, given that 'reading' the letter would not lead to correct responses in our paradigm (MacLeod, 1991). Our results are consistent with studies of normal perceivers showing that facilitation and interference rely on different mechanisms (Tzelgov et al., 1992).

In sum, immediately following rTMS of the right PPC, both participants showed a significant attenuation of interference normally induced by their synesthesia. We propose that right parietal rTMS produced a transient disruption of synesthetic color–form integration, thus reducing the conflict when the synesthetic photism did not correspond to the real color of the letter. These findings are consistent with evidence implicating the IPS/TOS in feature binding in normal perception (Donner et al., 2002; Friedman-Hill et al., 1995) and suggests that this region contributes to feature binding even when the perceived color is evoked by shape rather than wave-length (Robertson, 2003).

Table 1 Single-subject Reaction Times

	Participant E.F.			Participant C.P.		
	Neutral	Congruent	Incongruent	Neutral	Congruent	Incongruent
Right parietal						
Early phase						
Sham	476 ± 103	424 ± 77	546 ± 114	615 ± 161	574 ± 158	647 ± 186
rTMS	481 ± 88	423 ± 58	497 ± 96	550 ± 145	511 ± 118	535 ± 94
Late phase						
Sham	483 ± 86	453 ± 97	531 ± 92	548 ± 108	575 ± 169	597 ± 185
rTMS	509 ± 117	441 ± 80	570 ± 131	591 ± 166	546 ± 145	601 ± 184
Left parietal						
Early phase						
Sham	492 ± 120	434 ± 81	523 ± 116	503 ± 99	503 ± 104	544 ± 152
rTMS	469 ± 84	449 ± 93	530 ± 141	499 ± 118	471 ± 96	523 ± 134
Late phase						
Sham	496 ± 90	462 ± 94	529 ± 119	533 ± 113	521 ± 111	557 ± 132
rTMS	471 ± 95	462 ± 108	532 ± 133	495 ± 114	490 ± 103	536 ± 145
V1						
Early phase						
Sham	452 ± 76	419 ± 70	485 ± 91	591 ± 121	547 ± 141	611 ± 156
rTMS	440 ± 99	412 ± 62	488 ± 107	511 ± 106	486 ± 107	544 ± 144
Late phase						
Sham	423 ± 75	413 ± 64	514 ± 113	568 ± 117	556 ± 168	587 ± 150
rTMS	443 ± 98	418 ± 74	501 ± 84	524 ± 127	511 ± 132	529 ± 152

Shown are mean reaction times and standard deviations across each condition (neutral, congruent, or incongruent), phase (early, late), participant (E.F., C.P.) and each stimulation site (right parietal, left parietal, V1).

The present study supports the theory that feedback from a multimodal association region, like the parietal cortex, contributes to the perception of a synesthetic photism (Cohen-Kadosh & Henik, 2006; Sagiv et al., 2006; Robertson, 2003; Grossenbacher & Lovelace, 2001). Although this does not exclude the possibility that direct connections between fusiform regions also play a role in synesthesia (Ramachandran & Hubbard, 2001), it suggests that cross wiring between these regions is not always sufficient to bind the synesthetic percept to the inducing character.

An alternative explanation for our findings is that parietal TMS attenuates competition between perceptually related codes, similar to competition produced between the perceptually and conceptually related codes in the traditional Stroop task where the color of the word may be congruent or incongruent with the word itself. According to this view, parietal TMS would interfere with competition between the color word and color (traditional Stroop) as well as competition between two colors, one induced by wavelength and the other by the letter (synesthesia), rather than interfere with feature binding per se. Although imaging studies have associated parietal activity with Stroop tasks (MacLeod & MacDonald, 2000), it is unlikely that the parietal lobe plays a critical role in the competitive process underlying the traditional Stroop effect for several reasons. First, bilateral stimulation of the posterior parietal lobes does not influence the magnitude of Stroop interference or facilitation (Hayward, Goodwin, & Harmer, 2004).

Second, neuropsychological studies of patients with parietal lesions have demonstrated normal Stroop interference compared to controls. Interestingly, this effect has been reported in patients with either left, right, or bilateral infarcts (Vivas, Humphreys, & Fuentes, 2003; Robertson, Treisman, Friedman-Hill, & Grabowecky, 1997; Berti, Frassinetti, & Umilta, 1994), and these same patients may exhibit profound deficits in color–form binding (see Robertson, 2003). In contrast, alterations in Stroop performance have been associated with damage to the prefrontal cortex (Kato, 2001; Stuss, Floden, Alexander, Levine, & Katz, 2001).

Third, the three studies that have implicated the parietal lobe in color–grapheme synesthesia have not involved Stroop tasks, indicating that the parietal lobe's role in synesthesia is not dependent on response interference (Weiss et al., 2005; Elias et al., 2003; Rich et al., 2003). Together, these different lines of research strongly suggest that our effect is not due to response interference in general.

Behavioral and physiological evidence suggests that synesthesia is a heterogeneous phenomenon (Dixon & Smilek, 2005; Hubbard et al., 2005). These individual differences may be related to the degree of parietal involvement. One behavioral factor that may contribute to this heterogeneity is the difference between projectors, those who see the synesthetic photism in the world, and associators, those who see the photism in the mind's eye (Dixon et al., 2004). Although this factor has not been explored with respect to the degree of parietal involvement, one hypothesis to consider in future research is that synesthetes who show greater parietal involvement may tend to be 'projectors,' particularly when the synesthetic percept is tightly bound spatially to the inducing grapheme. Physiologically, the degree of parietal contribution among synesthetes may also be greater in individuals such as C.P., in whom the extent of early visual activation has been shown to be lesser (see Hubbard et al., 2005). Parietal participation in the synesthetic experience may correspond to the extent that attention is required to elicit the photism. The variability in the expression of color–grapheme synesthesia makes the examination of individual differences vital to our understanding of this fascinating phenomenon (Dixon & Smilek, 2005; Hubbard et al., 2005; Dixon et al., 2004). Our results have illuminated one of potentially several mechanisms responsible for synesthesia and are consistent with theories of how normal binding occurs within the human brain.

Future studies must examine the role of parietal binding mechanisms in other synesthetes, as well as investigate other parietal and temporal lobe regions that have been implicated in spatial attention and binding, such as the superior parietal cortex and the superior temporal sulcus, using both TMS and fMRI. In addition, single-pulse TMS will be able to elaborate on the temporal dynamics of the right PPC's involvement in synesthesia.

Acknowledgments

We thank Noam Sagiv for discussions and motivation that led to this project, Noam Sobel for comments on an early version of this manuscript, and Edward Hubbard for his constructive comments during the review process.

Reprint requests should be sent to Michael Esterman, Department of Psychology and Neuroscience Institute, University of California, Berkeley, CA, USA, or via e-mail: esterman@berkeley.edu.

Note

1   University of California, Berkeley, [2]Veterans Administration Medical Center, Martinez, CA.

References

Ashbridge, E., Walsh, V. and Cowey, A. (1997) Temporal aspects of visual search studied by transcranial magnetic stimulation. *Neuropsychologia, 35,* 1121–1131.

Berti, A., Frassinetti, F. and Umilta, C. (1994) Nonconscious reading? Evidence from neglect dyslexia. *Cortex, 30,* 181–197.

Chambers, J., Cleveland, W., Kleiner, B. and Tukey, P. (1983) *Graphical methods for data analysis (Wadsworth)* Boston: Duxbury Press.

Cohen-Kadosh, R. and Henik, A. (2006) Color congruity effect: Where do colors and numbers interact in synesthesia? *Cortex, 42,* 259–263.

Dixon, M.J. and Smilek, D. (2005) The importance of individual differences in grapheme–color synesthesia. *Neuron, 45,* 821–823.

Dixon, M.J., Smilek, D., Cudahy, C. and Merikle, P.M. (2000) Five plus two equals yellow. *Nature, 406,* 365.

Dixon, M.J., Smilek, D. and Merikle, P.M. (2004) Not all synaesthetes are created equal: Projector versus associator synaesthetes. *Cognitive, Affective, and Behavioral Neuroscience, 4,* 335–343.

Donner, T.H., Kettermann, A., Diesch, E., Ostendorf, F., Villringer, A. and Brandt, S.A. (2002) Visual feature and conjunction searches of equal difficulty engage only partially overlapping frontoparietal networks. *Neuroimage, 15,* 16–25.

Elias, L.J., Saucier, D.M., Hardie, C. and Sarty, G.E. (2003) Dissociating semantic and perceptual components of synaesthesia: Behavioral and functional neuroanatomical investigations. *Cognitive Brain Research, 16,* 232–237.

Epstein, C.M. and Davey, K.R. (2002) Iron-core coils for transcranial magnetic stimulation. *Journal of Clinical Neurophysiology, 19,* 376–381.

Friedman-Hill, S., Robertson, L. and Treisman, A. (1995) Parietal contributions to visual feature binding: Evidence from a patient with bilateral lesions. *Science, 269,* 853–855.

Grossenbacher, P.G. and Lovelace, C.T. (2001) Mechanisms of synesthesia: Cognitive and physiological constraints. *Trends in Cognitive Sciences, 5,* 36–41.

Hayward, G., Goodwin, G.M. and Harmer, C.J. (2004) The role of the anterior congulate cortex in the counting Stroop task. *Experimental Brain Research, 154,* 355–358.

Hubbard, E.M., Arman, A.C., Ramachandran, V.S. and Boynton, G.M. (2005) Individual differences among grapheme-color synesthetes: Brain-behavior correlations. *Neuron, 45,* 975–985.

Hubbard, E.M. and Ramachandran, V.S. (2005) Neurocognitive mechanisms of synesthesia. *Neuron, 48,* 509–520.

Kato, M. (2001) Prefrontal lobes and the attentional control: A neuropsychological study using modified Stroop test. *Rinsho Shinkeigaku, 41,* 1134–1136.

MacLeod, C.M. (1991) Half a century of research on the Stroop effect: An integrative review. *Psychological Bulletin, 109,* 163–203.

MacLeod, C.M. and MacDonald, P.A. (2000) Interdimensional interference in the Stroop effect: Uncovering the cognitive and neural anatomy of attention. *Trends in Cognitive Sciences, 4*, 383–391.

Manly, B. (1997) *Randomization, bootstrap and Monte Carlo methods in biology* (2nd ed.). New York: Chapman and Hall/CRC.

Mattingley, J.B., Rich, A.N., Yelland, G. and Bradshaw, J.L. (2001) Unconscious priming eliminates automatic binding of colour and alphanumeric form in synaesthesia. *Nature, 410*, 580–582.

Palmeri, T.J., Blake, R., Marois, R., Flanery, M.A. and Whetsell, W. (2002) The perceptual reality of synesthetic colors. *Proceedings of the National Academy of Sciences, U.S.A., 99*, 4127–4131.

Pascual-Leone, A., Tormos, J.M., Keenan, J., Tarazona, F., Canete, C. and Catala, M.D. (1998) Study and modulation of human cortical excitability with transcranial magnetic stimulation. *Journal of Clinical Neurophysiology, 15*, 333–343.

Ramachandran, V.S. and Hubbard, E.M. (2001) Psychophysical investigations into the neural basis of synaesthesia. *Proceedings of the Royal Society of London, Series B, Biological Sciences, 268*, 979–983.

Rich, A.N. and Mattingley, J.B. (2002) Anomalous perception in synaesthesia: A cognitive neuroscience perspective. *Nature Reviews, 3*, 43–52.

Rich, A.N., Puce, A., Syngeniotis, A., Williams, M.A., Howard, M.A., McGlone, F. and Mattingley, J.B. (2003) *Colour my brain: A functional neuroimaging study of color–graphemic synaesthesia.* Paper presented at the annual meeting of the Cognitive Neuroscience Society, New York, NY.

Robertson, L., Treisman, A., Friedman-Hill, S. and Grabowecky, M. (1997) The interaction of spatial and object pathways: Evidence from Balint's syndrome. *Journal of Cognitive Neuroscience, 9*, 295–317.

Robertson, L.C. (2003) Binding, spatial attention and perceptual awareness. *Nature Reviews Neuroscience, 4*, 93–102.

Sagiv, N., Heer, J. and Robertson, L.C. (2006) Does binding of synesthetic color to the evoking grapheme require attention? *Cortex, 42*, 232–242.

Smilek, D., Dixon, M.J. and Merikle, P.M. (2004) Binding of graphemes and synesthetic colors in color–graphemic synesthesia. In N. Sagiv & L. Robertson (Eds.), *Synesthesia: Perspectives from cognitive neuroscience.* New York: Oxford University Press.

Sperling, J.M., Prvulovic, D., Linden, D.E.J., Singer, W. and Stirn, A. (2006) Neuronal correlates of colour–graphemic synaesthesia: A fMRI study. *Cortex, 42*, 295–303.

Stuss, D.T., Floden, D., Alexander, M.P., Levine, B. and Katz, D. (2001) Stroop performance in focal lesion patients: Dissociation of processes and frontal lobe lesion location. *Neuropsychologia, 39*, 771–786.

Tzelgov, J., Henik, A. and Berger, J. (1992) Controlling Stroop effects by manipulating expectations for color words. *Memory & Cognition, 20*, 727–735.

Vivas, A.B., Humphreys, G.W. and Fuentes, L.J. (2003) Inhibitory processing following damage to the parietal lobe. *Neuropsychologia, 41*, 1531–1540.

Weiss, P.H., Zilles, K. and Fink, G.R. (2005) When visual perception causes feeling: Enhanced cross-modal processing in grapheme–color synesthesia. *Neuroimage, 28*, 859–868.

DESIGNING AND REPORTING EXPERIMENTS IN PSYCHOLOGY 3E

Peter Harris

This book will help undergraduate psychology students to write practical reports of experimental and other quantitative studies in psychology. It is designed to help with every stage of the report writing process including what to put in each section and recommendations for formatting and style. It also discusses how to design a study, including how to use and report relevant statistics. As such, the book acts both as an introduction and reference source to be used throughout an undergraduate course.

Key features of the new edition include:

- **New pedagogy**. Website icons within the text reference an enhanced website, **www.openup.co.uk/harris**, and 'Common Mistake' icons highlight common errors students should avoid. Statistics icons make reference to two key statistics books* where students can find more detailed information. A further icon indicates the presence of relevant commentary at the end of the book for more advanced students
- Discussion of how to write up different forms of quantitative study and report relevant statistics
- **Improved self-testing**. There are diagnostic questions (with answers at the end of the book) as well as fifty self-assessment questions within the text to aid student learning. Chapters in part two contain a list of methodological and statistical concepts covered that will help students to consolidate their knowledge
- A completely revised section on how to find and cite references plus current information on how to cite electronic references, incorporating the new APA guidelines
- Advice on the ethics of conducting research on the Internet

Contents: *Preface – To students – How to use this book – To tutors – Part one: Writing reports – Getting started – The introduction section – The method section – The results section – The discussion section – The title and abstract – References and appendices – Producing the final version of the report – Check list for report writing – What the marker's looking for – Mistakes to avoid – Part two: Design and statistics – Experiments, correlation and description – Basic experimental design – Statistics: significance testing – Statistics: effect size and power – More advanced experimental design – Commentary – Recommended reading – Appendix one: Confusing predictions from the null hypothesis with those from the experimental hypothesis – Appendix two: Randomizing – Appendix three: How to use tables of critical values of inferential statistics – Answers to SAQs – Answers to diagnostic questions – References – Index of concepts*

2008   308pp
978-0-335-22178-3 (Paperback)